The **Ultimate** Pit Boss Wood Pellet Smoker and Grill Cookbook

1000 Days Juicy and Flavorful Recipes to Help You Become the Undisputed Pitmaster of the Neighborhood

Table of Contents

INTRODUCTION

BEEF RECIPES

PORK RECIPES

LAMB RECIPES

CHICKEN RECIPES

VEGAN AND VEGETARIAN RECIPES

FISH AND SEAFOOD RECIPES

SNACK AND APPETIZERS RECIPES

DESSERT RECIPES

CONCLUSION

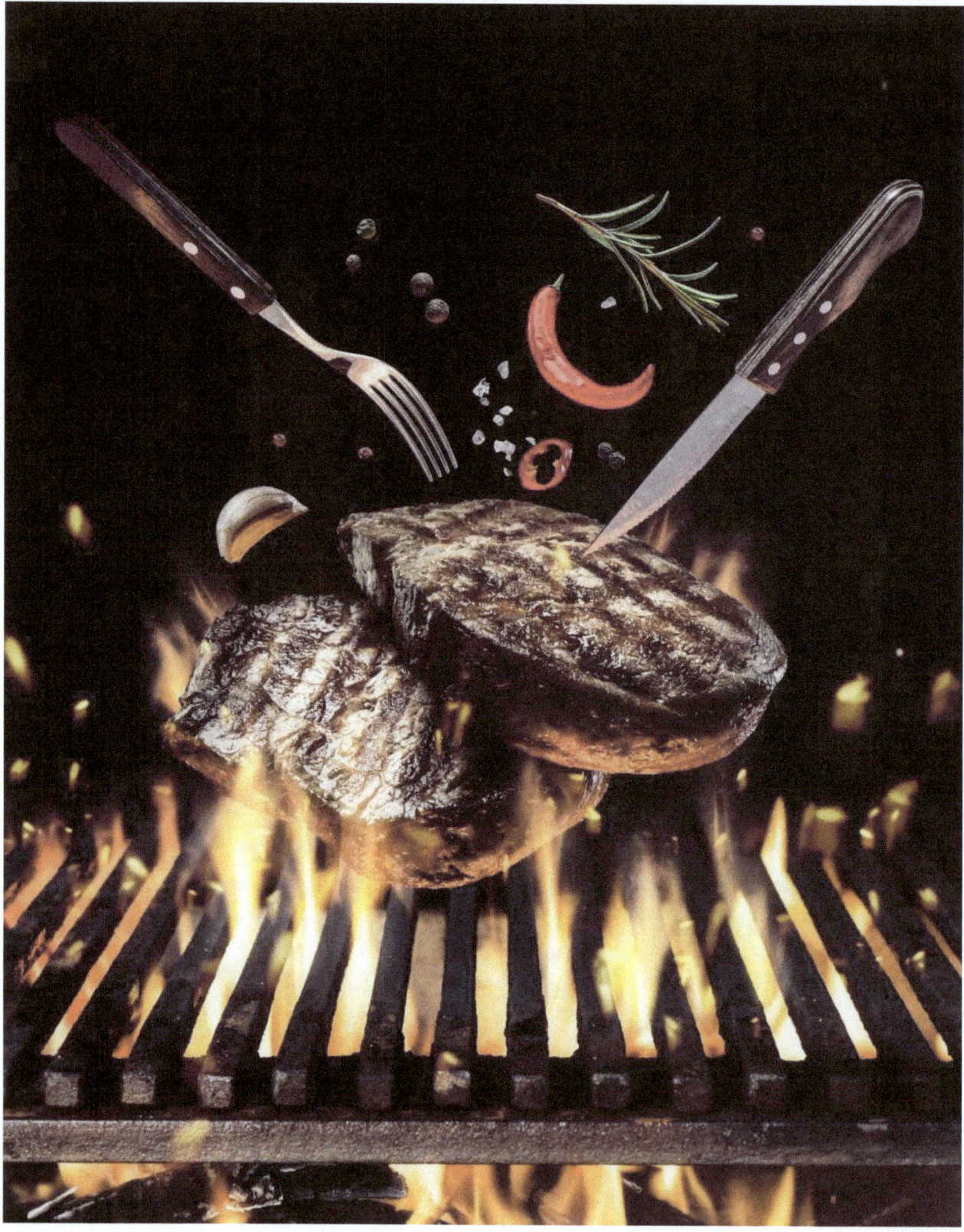

INTRODUCTION

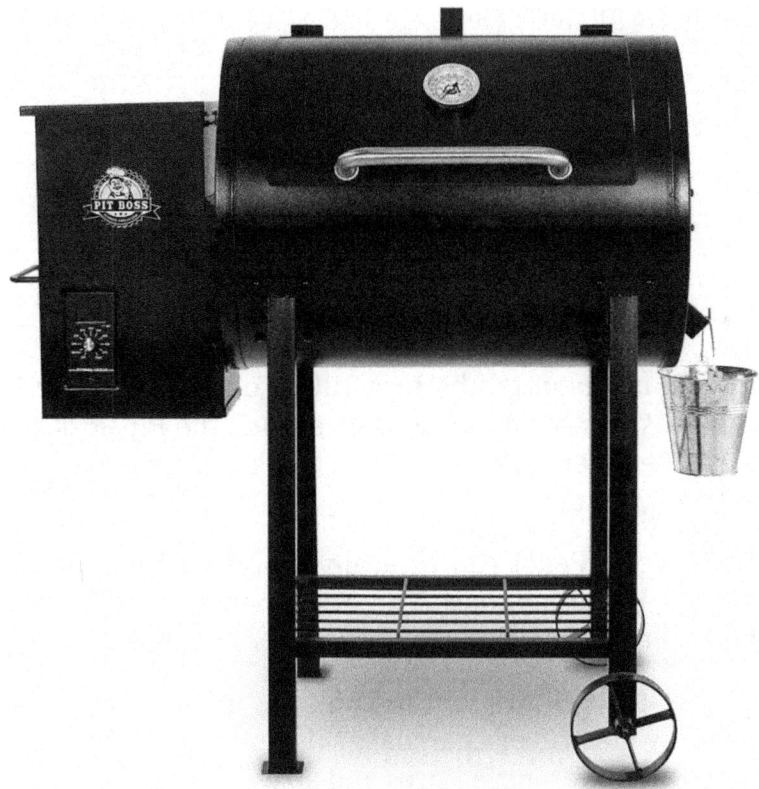

It's been almost a decade since I fell in love with grilled meat. I had attended my friend's wedding party when I was served with a delectable grilled lamb rib roast. The roast was very yummy, while the barbecue served alongside it greatly enhanced it. I swore to find the chef and master his grilling technique.

My grilling food journey has been filled with numerous twists and turns with relative success until I purchased my Pit Boss Wood Pellet Grill. I am not going to deny that I have had flavourful meats on charcoal and electric grills but have struggled to achieve a high-quality end product. With my Pit Boss Wood Pellet Grill, I have grilled and smoked food to my standards.

What is more, I have developed my grilling techniques through online classes and can attest that my grilling is now of a higher standard. Consequently, I am constantly entertaining my friends and family with mouth-watering delicious grilled food prepared in my Pit Boss Wood Pellet Grill.

In this book, I have compiled:

- What a Pit Boss Wood Pellet is

- How to use a Pit Boss Wood Pellet
- Grill skills to Pit Boss Pellet
- 1000 days delicious recipes

You can't stop now; the Grilling journey awaits you!

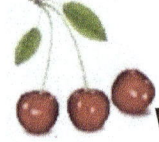

What is a Pit Boss Wood Pellet?

Pit Boss Wood Pellet Grill is one of the hottest BBQ products available in the market today. Whether outdoor enthusiasts or a competition-level chef, the Pit Boss Wood Pellet Grill pros appeal the same. Easy and efficient to use, it's a perfect kitchen gadget for anyone who wishes to enjoy classic grilled food right at home.

Otherwise, the Pit Boss Wood Pellet can clinically be defined as a BBQ pit that uses wood pellets to grill, smoke, bake, sear, or roast. The wood pellets come in different varieties that provide your food with unique flavours only hardwood can achieve.

The Pit Boss Wood Pellet Grill allows you to cook any food quickly and with the ultimate convenience unmatched by electric or charcoal grills. In addition, Pit Boss Wood Pellet Grills come in various brands with different features and sizes. Therefore, it's advisable to consult a buying guide before you make a purchase.

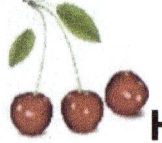

How to use a Pit Boss Wood Pellet?

If you have never used a Pit Boss Wood Pellet Grill before, it can appear to be intimidating. They differ from charcoal, electric, or gas grills but are super easy to use. Let's have an overview of how to use them.

- First things first, clean any leftover ashes in the fire pot from the previous cooking. The fire pot is where the wood pellets and ash residue are found.
- Plugin the grill into a power source and set the temperature dial to smoke on the control panel. Press the power button.
- You will hear the fan and the auger move. The auger is the tunnel that feeds the fire pot. You may control the amount of pellets by using the Prime feature on the control panel.

- Put your hand over the fire pot without touching it to ensure there is airflow. You should also smell the ignitor and feel the air getting warm. Turn off the grill.
- Open the lid and add wood pellets to the hopper. A hopper is a large storage container attached to the grill that holds the pellets before being fed to the cooking chamber.
- Turn on the grill and set to smoke while holding the Prime button until you see pellets fall in the fire pot.
- Turn the wood pellet grill to high temperature and close the lid. Preheating the grill will take about 15 minutes.
- Place the food on the desired cooking component.
- **Top shelf**

This is mainly used as an additional cooking space. You may also cook food that requires low heat and longer times to cook.

- **Bottom cooking surface**

This is the main cooking area. It has removable grill grates and varies depending on the model

- **Flame broiler**

The flame broiler is used for flame broiling or for using cast-iron pans for cooking your food.

- Close the lid and let your Pit Boss Wood pallet do its thing.
- Once the food is cooked, remove the food from the grill and conduct the burn-off procedure- Close the lid, turn it to the highest setting and let it run for about 10 minutes. The burn-off process reduces the risk of a grease fire in the following cooking.

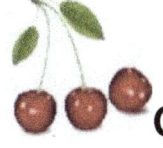

Grill skills to Pit Boss Pellet

1. Ensure to wash your grill after every use. Failure to do so may ruin your grill. More to it, residue food from last cooking may give your current food a foul smell.
2. Test different flavours of pellets such as mesquite, hickory, apple wood, and many more. Your choice of pellets will play a massive role in the taste of food.
3. When switching from high to low temperature, open the lid until the temperature is close to your desired temperature. This ensures the fire doesn't go out and speeds up the process.
4. Cook for longer with lower temperatures to infuse more smoke flavour in your foods.

5. Do not overcrowd the food for proper heat flow and shorter cooking periods. Overcrowded food will require more time to cook.
6. When cooking for long periods, use a water pan to add humidity and stabilize heat.
7. Do not open the lid when smoking. Doing so will cause a temperature drop and interfere with the smoking process.
8. Invest in long-handled tongs and a spatula for turning meats. Do not use forks or any sharp objects. Poking the meat will allow juices to escape.

BEEF RECIPES

Smoked Cowboy Tri-Tip

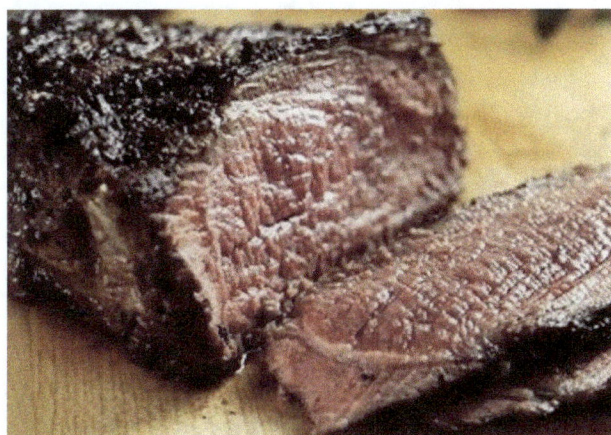

Prep Time: 15 minutes
Cook Time: 4 hours
Serves: 6

Ingredients

- 3 Pounds tri-tip
- ⅛ cup coffee, grounded
- ¼ cup beef rub

Preparation:

1. Fire up your Pit Boss Wood Pellet Grill to 180 degrees F with the lid closed for 15 minutes.
2. Rub the meat with coffee and beef rub until well coated.
3. Place the meat on the grill grates and smoke for 3 hours.
4. Remove the meat and increase the heat to 300 degrees F.
5. Double wrap the meat and place it on the grill. Let cook for 45 minutes or until the internal temperature reaches 130 degrees F.
6. Let the meat rest before slicing and serving.

Serving suggestion: serve the cowboy tri-tip with sautéed veggies

Variation Tip: use dried herbs and spice of choice in place of beef rub

Nutrition-Per Serving:

Calories 421 | Fat 22g | Sodium 1640mg | Carbs 1g | Fiber 0g | Sugar 1g | Protein 50g

Teriyaki Beef Jerky

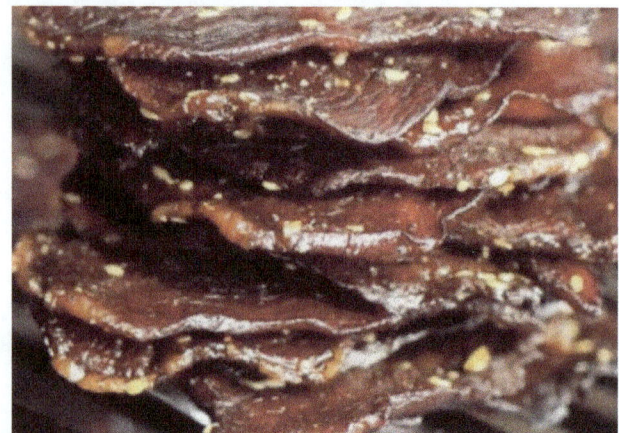

Prep Time: 15 minutes
Cook Time: 4 hours
Serves: 8

Ingredients:

- 3 cups soy sauce
- 2 cups brown sugar
- 3 garlic cloves
- 1-inch ginger, diced finely
- 1 tablespoon sesame oil
- 4 Pounds skirt steak

Preparation:

1. Add all ingredients to a blender except for the steak. Blend until smooth.
2. Trim any excess fat from the steak and slice into ¼ inch slices.
3. Add the marinade and the steak in a ziplock bag, mix well and place in the fridge overnight.
4. Fire up your Pit Boss Wood Pellet Grill to 160 degrees F for 5 minutes. Arrange the steak on the grill grate without overlapping.
5. Cook for 5 minutes. Remove from the grill and let it cool before serving. Enjoy.

Serving suggestion: serve beef jerky with sunflower seeds and teriyaki sauce

Variation Tip: use ginger and low sodium soy sauce

Nutrition-Per Serving:
Calories 670 | Fat 25g |Sodium 5573 mg | Carbs43 g | Fiber 0.8g | Sugar 37g | Protein 70g

Grilled Butter Busted Rib-Eye

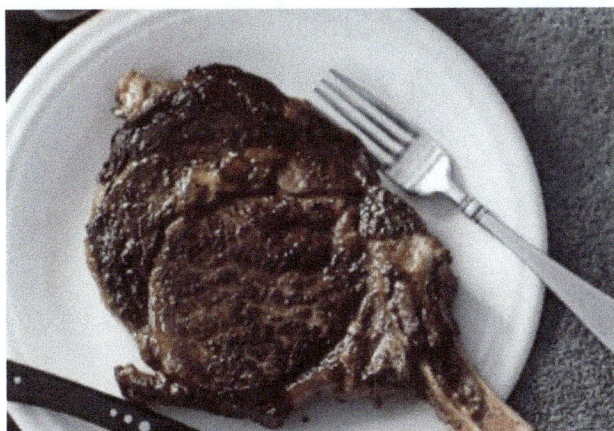

Prep Time: 5 minutes
Cook Time: 15 minutes
Serves: 2

Ingredients:

- 2 thickly cut rib-eye steaks
- Salt to taste
- Pepper to taste
- 4 tablespoons butter

Preparation:

1. Season the steak with salt and pepper to taste. Let marinate for 20 minutes.
2. Preheat the Pit Boss Wood Pellet Grill to 500 degrees F for 15 minutes with the lid closed.
3. Place a cast-iron pan on the grill grate and let preheat.
4. Place the steak on the grill grate and let cook for 5 minutes.
5. Place butter on the hot pan then transfers the steak to the pan.
6. Cook the steak while basting it with butter every 5 minute. Cook the steak until the internal temperature reaches 125 degrees F.
7. Remove the steak from the grill and let rest for 10 minutes before serving. Enjoy.

Serving suggestion: serve the rib eye with sautéed veggies

Variation Tip: use dried herbs and spice of choice in place of beef rub

Nutrition-Per Serving:
Calories 304 | Fat 25g |Sodium 1221mg | Carbs 1g | Fiber 0g | Sugar 0g | Protein 42g

Pit Boss Wood Pellet Grill Smoked Brisket

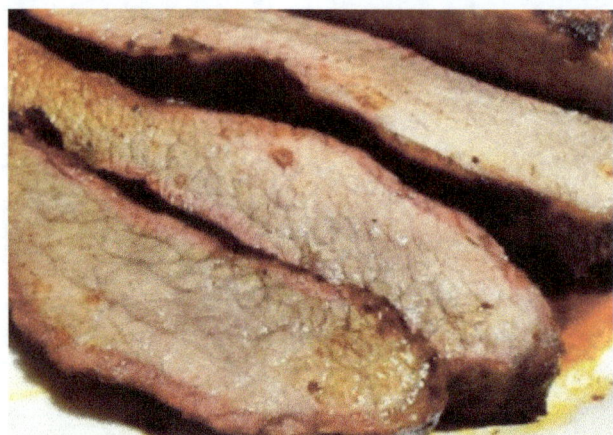

Prep Time: 15 minutes
Cook Time: 9 hours
Serves: 6

Ingredients:

- 1½ tablespoons garlic powder
- 1½ tablespoons onion powder
- 1½ tablespoons paprika
- 1½ tablespoons chili powder
- ¼ cup kosher salt
- ¼ cup black pepper
- 12 Pounds brisket
- 1½ cup beef broth

Preparation:

1. Fire up your Pit Boss Wood Pellet Grill to 225 degrees F for 15 minutes with the lid closed.
2. Mix all ingredients in a mixing bowl except the brisket and broth.
3. Season the brisket generously with the rub then place it on the grill grates with the fat side down.
4. Grill it for 6 hours or until the internal temperature reaches 160 degrees F.
5. Remove the meat from the grill and double wrap it with aluminium foil. Add the broth to the foil.
6. Return it to the grill and cook for an additional 3 hours or until the internal temperature reaches 204 degrees F.
7. Remove from the grill, unwrap it and let rest for 15 minutes before serving. Enjoy.

Serving suggestion: serve the brisket alongside rice and sauteed broccoli

Variation Tip: use beef rub and spray apple juice occasionally

Nutrition-Per Serving:
Calories 3530 | Fat 287g |Sodium 5481mg | Carbs 6g | Fiber 2g | Sugar 2g | Protein 215g

Smoked Deli Style Beef Roast

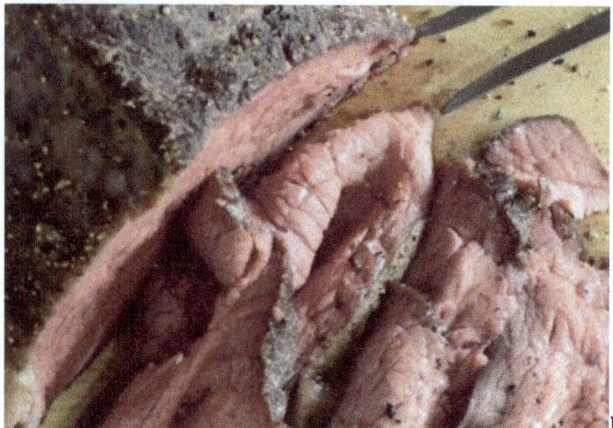

Prep Time: 15 minutes
Cook Time: 4 hours
Serves: 10

Ingredients:

- 4 Pounds beef roast
- 1 tablespoon coconut oil
- ¼ tablespoons garlic powder
- ¼ tablespoons onion powder
- ¼ tablespoons thyme
- ¼ tablespoons oregano
- ½ tablespoons paprika
- ½ tablespoons salt
- ½ tablespoons black pepper

Preparation:

1. Combine all the dry ingredients until well combined.
2. Roll the roast in the rub and coat well using your hands.
3. Preheat your Pit Boss Wood Pellet Grill to 185 degrees F with the lid closed
4. Smoke the meat for 4 hours or until the internal temperature reaches 140 degrees F.
5. Remove the meat from the grill and let cool for 10 minutes before slicing and serving.

Serving suggestion: Serve the beef roast n a sandwich with caramelized onions

Variation Tip: use Dijon mustard and brown sugar

Nutrition-Per Serving:
Calories 352 | Fat 26g |Sodium 469mg | Carbs 2g | Fiber 0.3g | Sugar 0.2g | Protein 55g

Supper Grilled Beef Roast

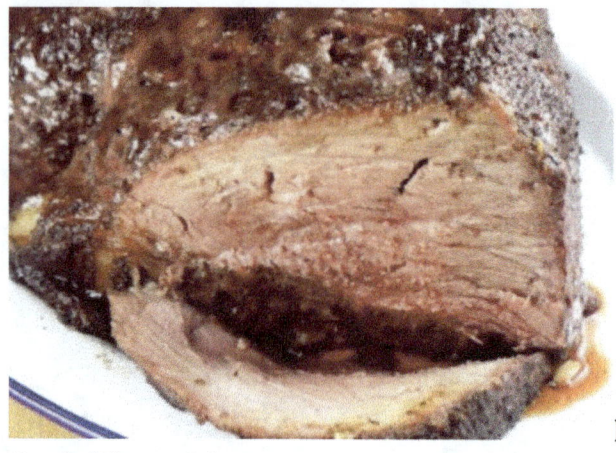

Prep Time: 5 minutes
Cook Time: 3 hours
Serves: 6

Ingredients:

- 3 Pounds beef top round
- 3 tablespoons vegetable oil
- Rib rub of choice
- 2 cups beef broth
- 1 russet potato, sliced into 1-inch pieces
- 2 carrots, sliced into 1-inch pieces
- 2 celery stalks, sliced into 1-inch pieces
- 1 onion, sliced into 1-inch pieces
- 2 thyme sprigs

Preparation:

1. Rub the beef with oil and place it on a lack in a pan.
2. Rub the meat well then pour the beef broth into the pan.
3. Fire up your Pit Boss Wood Pellet Grill to 500 degrees F with the lid closed for 15 minutes.
4. Place the pan on the grill grates and cook for 25 minutes or until the outside is well seared.
5. Reduce heat to 225 degrees F then add the vegetables with the thyme sprig to the pan.
6. Cover the pan with aluminium foil and cook for 3 hours or until the meat's internal temperature reaches 135 degrees F.
7. Remove the pan from the grill and let rest for 10 minutes before slicing the beef and serving.

8. Serve the beef with pan juices and vegetables. Enjoy.

Serving suggestion: Serve the beef roast alongside rice or mashed potatoes

Variation Tip: use Worcestershire sauce and prime rib rub

Nutrition-Per Serving:
Calories 579 | Fat 29g | Sodium 410mg | Carbs 4g | Fiber 1g | Sugar 2g | Protein 70g

Smoked Ribeye Steak

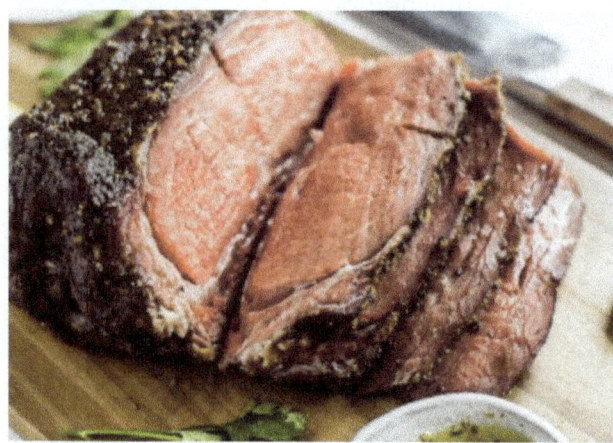

Prep Time: 15 minutes
Cook Time: 35 minutes
Serves: 1

Ingredients:

- ½ Pounds ribeye steak
- Steak rubs of choice

Preparation:

1. Preheat your Pit Boss Wood Pellet Grill to 180 degrees F for 30 minutes.
2. Sprinkle the steak with rub and smoke it in the grill for 25 minutes.
3. Remove the steak from the grill and increase the temperature to 400 degrees F.
4. Sear each side of the steak for 5 minutes or until the internal temperature reaches 125 degrees F.
5. Wrap the steak with aluminium foil and let sit for 10 minutes. Slice and serve.

Serving suggestion: Serve the ribeye steak alongside grilled carrots

Variation Tip: use dried herbs and spices of choice

Nutrition-Per Serving:
Calories 756 | Fat 37g |Sodium 1496mg | Carbs 65g | Fiber 3g | Sugar 4g | Protein 36g

Grilled Beef Jerky

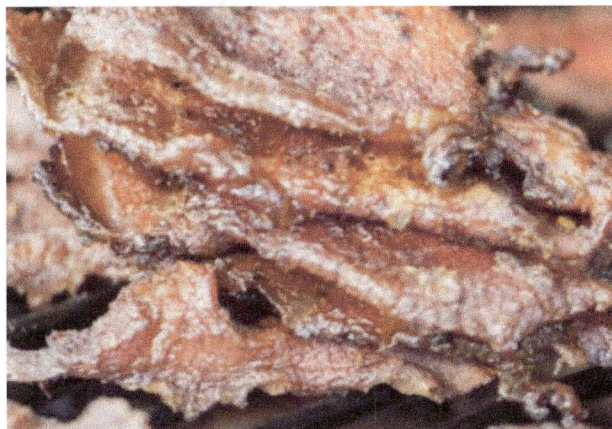

Prep Time: 15 minutes
Cook Time: 5 hours
Serves: 10

Ingredients:

- 3 Pounds sirloin steaks, cut into ¼ -inch slices
- 2 cups soy sauce
- ½ cup brown sugar
- 1 cup pineapple juice
- 2 tablespoons sriracha
- 2 tablespoons red pepper flake
- 2 tablespoons hoisin
- 2 tablespoons onion powder
- 2 tablespoons rice wine vinegar
- 2 tablespoons garlic cloves, minced

Preparation:

1. Add all the ingredients in a resealable bag and shake to mix. Marinate the beef for 6 hours in the refrigerator.
2. Remove the beef from the refrigerator 1 hour before cooking.
3. Fire up the Pit Boss Wood Pellet Grill to 375 degrees F.
4. Layer the beef on the grill leaving space between all the pieces.
5. Grill the beef jerky for 5 hours, turning them after 2 hours of grilling.
6. Serve and enjoy.

Serving suggestion: Serve the jerky with butter sauce

Variation Tip: Use dried herbs and prime meat

Nutrition-Per Serving:

Calories 309 | Fat 3g | Sodium 2832mg | Carbs 20g | Fiber 1g | Sugar 15g | Protein 34g

Smoked and Pulled Beef

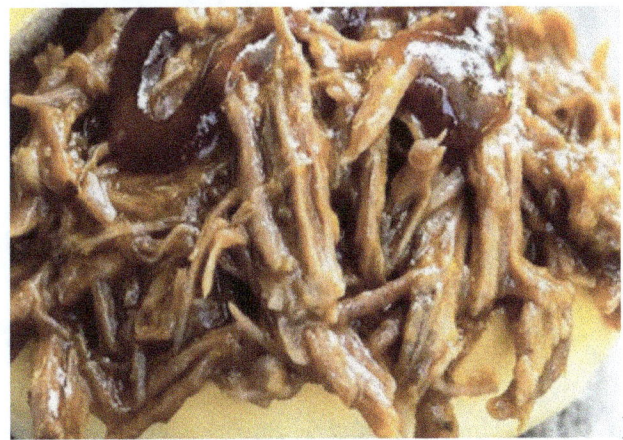

Prep Time: 15minutes
Cook Time: 5 hours
Serves: 6

Ingredients:

- 3 Pounds beef sirloin tip roast
- ½ cup BBQ dry rub
- 2 cans of amber beer
- 1 bottle barbecue sauce
- 6 buns

Preparation:

1. Trim excess fat from the beef roast and coat it with the BBQ dry rub.
2. Fire up your Pit Boss wood pellet grill to 180 degrees F.
3. Place the beef roast on the grill and smoke for 3 hours turning it after every 1 hour.
4. Place the beef in a braising pan and add the beer. Braise the beef on the grill for 4 hours.
5. Remove the beef from the pan and shred it with a fork.
6. Return the shredded beef into the pan and stir in the barbecue sauce.
7. Serve and enjoy.

Serving suggestion: Serve the pulled beef with pasta

Variation Tip: Use dried herbs and prime meat

Nutrition-Per Serving:
Calories 829 | Fat 46g |Sodium 181mg | Carbs 4g | Fiber 0g | Sugar 0g | Protein 86g

Reverse Seared Flank Steak

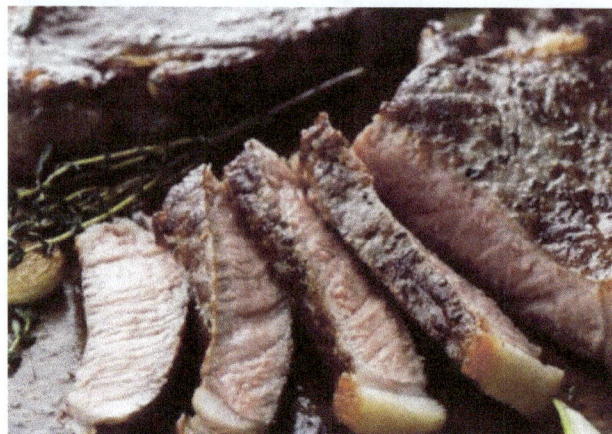

Prep Time: 10 minutes
Cook Time: 20 minutes
Serves: 6

Ingredients:

- 1 tablespoon salt
- ½ tablespoons onion powder
- ¼ tablespoons garlic powder
- ½ tablespoons coarsely ground black pepper
- 3 Pounds flank steak
- Basil for garnishing

Preparation:

1. In a bowl, mix salt, onion powder, garlic powder, and black pepper.
2. Rub the steak with the seasoning mixture.
3. Preheat your Pit Boss Wood Pellet Grill to 225 degrees F.
4. Place the steak on the grill and cook for about 4 hours until the steak is 125 degrees F.
5. Remove the steak from the grill and crank up the grill temperature to 500 degrees F.
6. Place the steak on the grill and grill for 3 minutes on each side.
7. Serve and enjoy.

Serving suggestion: Serve the flank steak with a pat of butter

Variation Tip: Use fresh onion and crushed/ minced garlic

Nutrition-Per Serving:
Calories 112 | Fat 5g |Sodium 737mg | Carbs 1g | Fiber 0g | Sugar 0g | Protein 16g

Pit Boss Wood Pellet Smoked Brisket

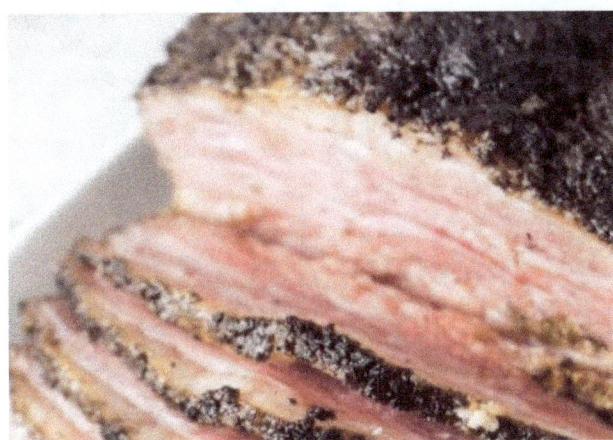

Prep Time: 15 minutes
Cook Time: 12 minutes
Serves: 6

Ingredients:

- 1 tablespoon Worcestershire sauce
- 1 tablespoon brisket dry rub
- 4 Pounds flat cut brisket
- 1 cup beef broth

Preparation:

1. In a bowl mix the Worcestershire sauce and the brisket dry rub. Rub the seasoning mixture onto the brisket.
2. Set the wood pellet grill to 180 degrees F.
3. Place the brisket on the grill and smoke for 7 hours.
4. Tightly wrap the brisket with double-wall aluminium foil and add the broth.
5. Crank the grill temperature to 225 degrees F and grill the brisket for 5 hours.
6. Let the brisket rest for 30 minutes before slicing.
7. Serve and enjoy.

Serving suggestion: Serve the smoked brisket with sautéed broccoli and peppers.

Variation Tip: omit Worcestershire sauce and use homemade rub

Nutrition-Per Serving:
Calories 454 | Fat 18g |Sodium 2804mg | Carbs 0.7g | Fiber 0g | Sugar 0.6g | Protein 41g

Grilled Butter Basted Porterhouse Steak

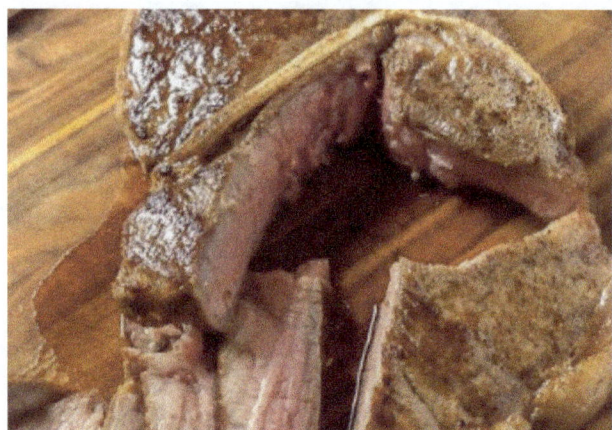

Prep Time: 5 minutes
Cook Time: 40 minutes
Serves: 2

Ingredients:

- 4 tablespoons melted butter
- 2 tablespoons Worcestershire sauce
- 2 tablespoons Dijon mustard
- 20 Ounce porterhouse steaks cut into 1-inch thick pieces
- 1 tablespoon prime rib rub
- 1 rosemary sprig

Preparation:

1. Preheat your Pit Boss Wood Pellet Grill to 225 degrees F.
2. In a bowl whisk the butter, Worcestershire sauce, and mustard.
3. Brush the steak with the seasoning mixture then coat with the prime rib rub.
4. Layer the steak on the grill and cook for 30 minutes.
5. Remove the steak from the grill and raise the grill temperature to 500 degrees F.
6. Place the steak on the grill and grill for 3 minutes on each side.
7. Let the steak rest for 3 minutes before slicing.
8. Garnish the steak with rosemary and serve.

Serving suggestion: Serve the butter-basted porterhouse steak with some green salad

Variation Tip: Add a splash of Guinness for a coffee hint

Nutrition-Per Serving:
Calories 869 | Fat 67g |Sodium 702mg | Carbs 4g | Fiber 0.5g | Sugar 3.1g | Protein 60g

Cocoa Crusted Grilled Flank Steak

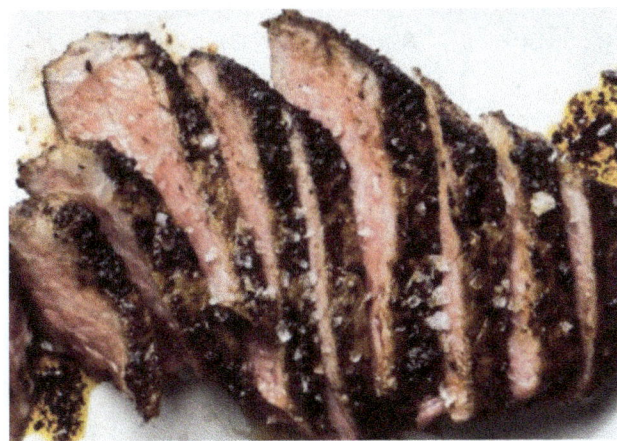

Prep Time: 15 minutes
Cook Time: 10 minutes
Serves: 6

Ingredients:

- 1 tablespoon cocoa powder
- 2 tablespoons chili powder
- 1 tablespoon chipotle chile powder
- ½ tablespoons garlic powder
- ½ tablespoons onion powder
- 1½ tablespoons brown sugar
- 1 tablespoon kosher salt
- ½ tablespoons black pepper
- 1 tablespoon cumin
- 1 tablespoon smoked paprika
- 3 Pounds flank steak
- 2 tablespoons oil

Preparation:

1. In a bowl mix cocoa powder, chili powder, chipotle chile powder, garlic powder, onion powder, brown sugar, salt, black pepper, cumin, and smoked paprika.
2. Brush the steak with oil then rub it with the cocoa mixture.
3. Fire up your Pit Boss Wood Pellet Grill to 500 degrees F.
4. Cook the steak for about 5 minutes on each side.
5. Let the steak rest for 10 minutes before slicing.
6. Serve and enjoy.

Serving suggestion: Serve this Frank steak in tacos

Variation Tip: reduce the chili and cumin if you don't want it too spicy.

Nutrition-Per Serving:

Calories 335 | Fat 12g |Sodium 1319mg | Carbs 7g | Fiber 2g | Sugar 3g | Protein 50g

Prime Rib Roast

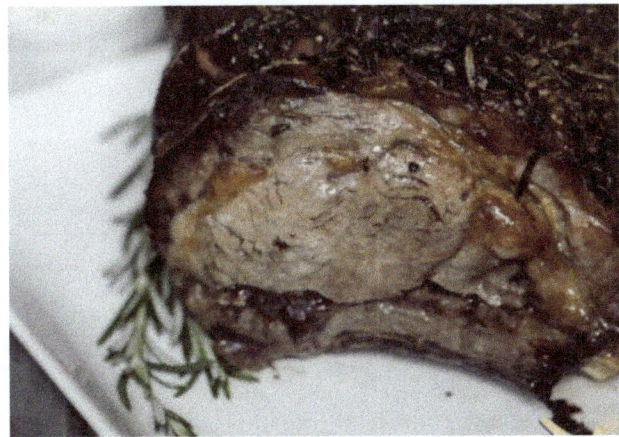

Prep Time: 5 minutes
Cook Time: 4 hours
Serves: 8

Ingredients:

- 5 bone prime rib roast
- 2 tablespoons prime rib rub

Preparation:

1. Coat the rib roast with prime rib rub and marinate it in a plastic wrap for 24 hours.
2. Fire up your Pit Boss Wood Pellet Grill to 500 degrees F.
3. Place the rib on the grill grate with the fat side up. Grill the rib for 30 minutes.
4. Reduce the grill temperature to 300 degrees F and cook for about 4 hours.
5. Let the rib roast rest for 30 minutes before carving.
6. Serve and enjoy.

Serving suggestion: Serve this rib roast with pasta or rice and roasted onions.

Variation Tip: put a certain amount of rib if you don't eat too much

Nutrition-Per Serving:
Calories 699 | Fat 60g | Sodium 1469mg | Carbs 1g | Fiber 1g | Sugar 2g | Protein 38g

PORK RECIPES

Grilled Blackened Pork Chops

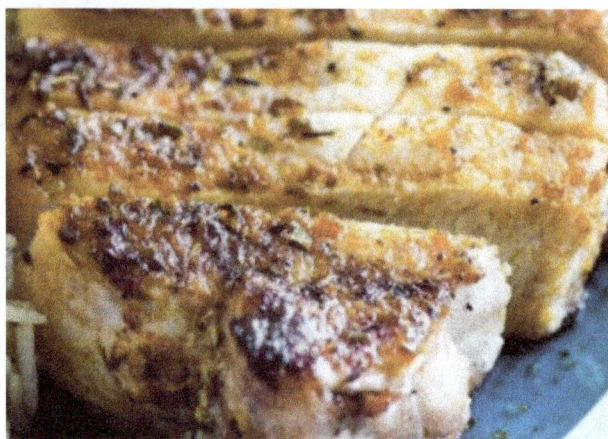

Prep Time: 7 minutes
Cook Time: 20 minutes
Serves: 6

Ingredients:

- 6 pork chops
- ¼ cup blackening seasoning of choice
- Salt and pepper to taste

Preparation:

1. Fire up your wood pellet to 375 degrees F.
2. Meanwhile, season the pork chops with seasoning, salt, and pepper.
3. Place the chops in the grill and cook for 7 minutes per side with the lid closed.
4. The chops should have an internal temperature of 140 degrees F.
5. Remove the chops from the grill and let them rest for 10 minutes before serving.
6. Slice and serve.

Serving suggestion: Serve the pork chops with rice and sautéed broccoli

Variation Tip: use BBQ rub, garlic powder, and onion powder in place of blackening seasoning.

Nutrition-Per Serving:
Calories 333 | Fat 17g |Sodium 3175mg | Carbs 1g | Fiber 1g | Sugar 0g | Protein 41g

Grilled Pineapple Pork Sliders

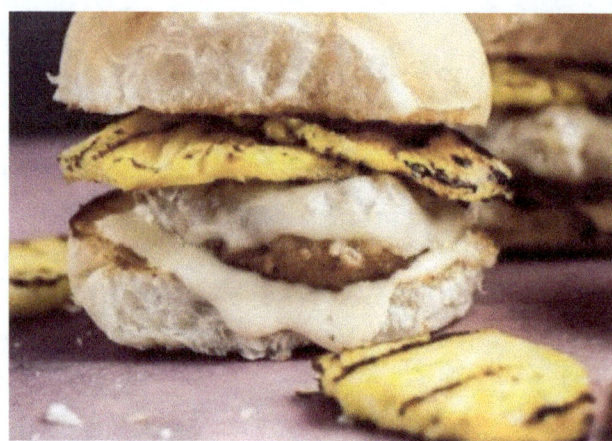

Prep Time: 20 minutes
Cook Time: 20 minutes
Serves: 6

Ingredients:

- 1½ tablespoons salt
- 1 tablespoon onion powder
- 1 tablespoon paprika
- ½ tablespoons garlic powder
- ½ tablespoons cayenne pepper1½ pork tenderloin
- 1 can pineapple rings
- 1 package Hawaiian rolls
- 8 ounce teriyaki sauce
- Lettuce leaves for serving

Preparation:

1. Add all dry ingredients to a mixing bowl and mix well to make a rub.
2. Apply the paprika on the tenderloin until well coated.
3. Fire up your Pit Boss Wood Pellet Grill to 325 degrees F.
4. Place the tenderloin on the grill and cook while the lid is closed while turning occasionally after every 4 minutes until the internal temperature reaches 145 degrees F.
5. While the pork is cooking, place the pineapple rings on the grill. flip the rings once they have brown marks on them.
6. Cut the rolls in halves and place them on the grill alongside tenderloin and pineapple rings. Let them cook until they have grill marks and are toasty brown.

7. Assemble the sliders by putting the bottom roll followed by the lettuce leaf, tenderloin, pineapple ring, teriyaki sauce, and the top roll.
8. Serve and enjoy.

Serving suggestion: Serve the pork sliders alongside potato chips and tomato sauce.

Variation Tip: use regular buns and some veggies such as onions and lettuce

Nutrition-Per Serving:
Calories 243 | Fat 5g |Sodium 2447 mg | Carbs 15g | Fiber 1g | Sugar 10g | Protein 33g

Grilled Pork Tenderloin with Fresh herb sauce

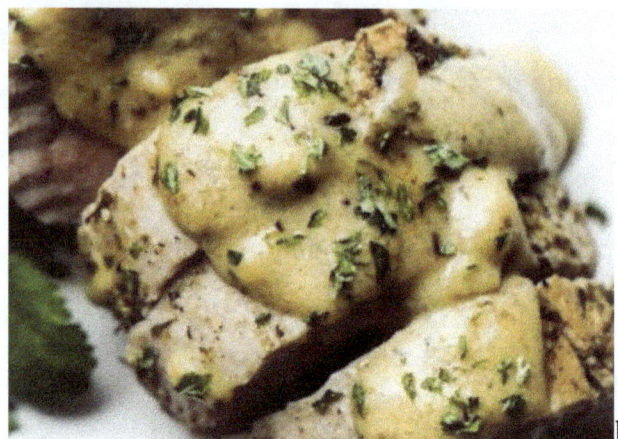

Prep Time: 10 minutes
Cook Time: 15 minutes
Serves: 4

Ingredients:

Pork
- 1 pork tenderloin
- BBQ seasoning

Fresh Herb sauce
- ½ handful flat-leaf parsley, fresh
- 1 handful basil, fresh
- ¼ tablespoons garlic powder
- ⅓ cup oil
- ½ tablespoons salt

Preparation:

1. Fire up your Pit Boss Wood Pellet Grill to medium heat.
2. Remove silver skin from the tenderloin and pat it dry with a paper towel.
3. Coat the tenderloin generously with BBQ seasoning. Cook on the grill while turning it frequently for 15 minutes or until the internal temperature reaches 140 degrees F.
4. Remove from the grill and let rest for 10 minutes.
5. Meanwhile, add all the herb sauce ingredients to a food processor and pulse a few times.
6. Slice the pork and serve with the herb sauce. Enjoy.

Serving suggestion: Serve the pork tenderloin with cheesy orzo or grilled asparagus

Variation Tip: use herbs of choice to make the sauce

Nutrition-Per Serving:
Calories 300 | Fat 22g |Sodium 791 mg | Carbs 13g | Fiber 1g | Sugar 10g | Protein 14g

Pit Boss Wood Pellet Grill Pork Tacos

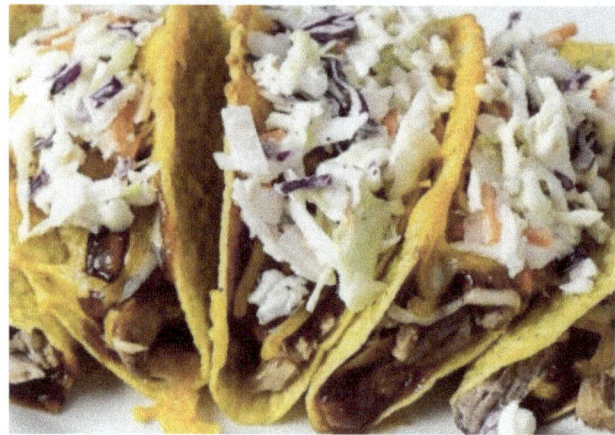

Prep Time: 15 minutes
Cook Time: 6 hours
Serves: 8

Ingredients:

- 3 tablespoons brown sugar
- 1 tablespoon salt
- 1 tablespoon garlic powder
- 1 tablespoon paprika
- 1 tablespoon onion powder
- ¼ tablespoons cumin
- 1 tablespoon cayenne pepper
- 5 pounds pork shoulder roast

Preparation:

1. Add all ingredients in a mixing bowl except pork to make a dry rub.
2. Rub the pork with the rub until well coated.
3. Place the pork in the Pit Boss Wood Pellet Grill at 250 degrees F for 6 hours or until the internal temperature is 190 degrees F.
4. Let the pork rest for 10 minutes before shredding and serving in tacos. Enjoy.

Serving suggestion: Serve with taco fixings of choice like peppers, parsley, and onions

Variation Tip: Don't shred and serve it alongside cooked white rice

Nutrition-Per Serving:
Calories 566 | Fat 42g |Sodium 660 mg | Carbs 4g | Fiber 0g | Sugar 2g | Protein 44g

Grilled Pulled pork

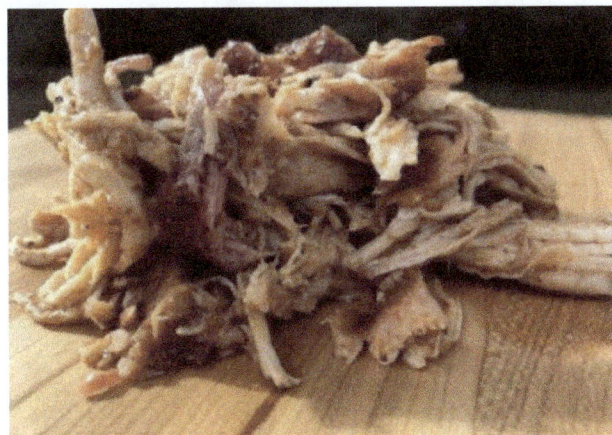

Prep Time: 15 minutes
Cook Time: 12 hours
Serves: 12

Ingredients:

- 8 Pounds pork shoulder roast
- Bbq rub
- 3 cups hard apple cider

Preparation:

1. Preheat your Pit Boss Wood Pellet Grill to 180 degrees F and set it to smoke.
2. Meanwhile, rub the roast with BBQ rub on all sides then place it on the grill grates.
3. Smoke the pork for 5 hours while flipping it after every hour.
4. Increase the heat to 225 degrees F and cook for an additional 3 hours. Transfer the pork to a foil pan and add cider to the pan.
5. Cook until the internal temperature of the meat reaches 200 degrees F
6. Remove the pork from the grill and tent it for 1 hour with a foil. Shred with a fork and serve.

Serving suggestion: Serve the pulled pork with potato chip nachos

Variation Tip: use regular apple juice in place of apple cider

Nutrition-Per Serving:
Calories 912 | Fat 65g |Sodium 208 mg | Carbs 7g | Fiber 0g | Sugar 6g | Protein 70g

Pit Boss Wood Pellet Grilled Pork Ribs

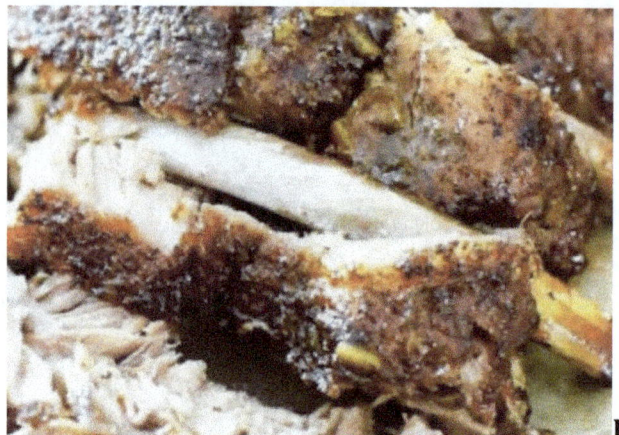

Prep Time: 10 minutes
Cook Time: 11 hours
Serves: 4

Ingredients:

- 2 racks pork ribs
- 1 cup BBQ rub
- 24 Ounce hard apple cider
- 1 cup dark brown sugar
- 2 batches BBQ sauce

Preparation:

1. Fire up your Pit Bos Wood Pellet Grill to 180 degrees F.
2. Meanwhile, remove the membrane from the ribs and coat with BBQ rub.
3. Smoke the ribs for 5 hours. Transfer the ribs to a baking pan and pour apple cider into the pan.
4. Rub the ribs with sugar and cover the pan with foil.
5. Place the pan on the grill and cook for an additional 4 hours.
6. Place the ribs directly on the grill grates and increase the temperature to 300 degrees F.
7. Brush BBQ sauce on the ribs regularly as you cook them for an additional 1 hour. Serve and enjoy.

Serving suggestion: Serve pork ribs with a fresh salad of choice

Variation Tip: experiment with a different pre-made rub or homemade rub

Nutrition-Per Serving:
Calories 1073 | Fat 42g | Sodium 1663 mg | Carbs 111g | Fiber 3g | Sugar 99g | Protein 61g

Smoked Pork Ribs

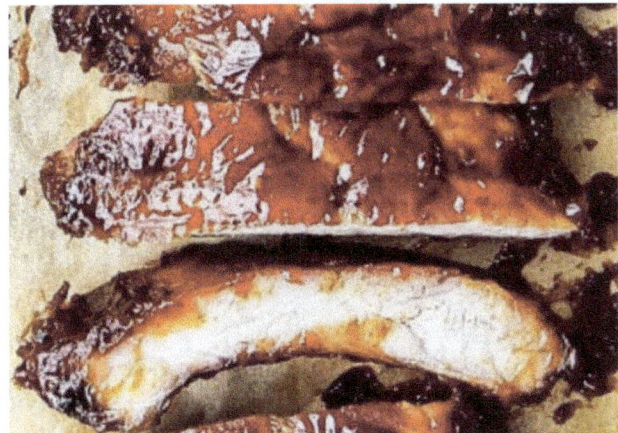

Prep Time: 15 minutes
Cook Time: 4 hours 45 minutes
Serves: 12

Ingredients:

- 3 racks baby back ribs
- ¾ cup dry rib rub
- ¾ cup BBQ sauce

Preparation:

1. Trim excess fat from the backside of the ribs and peel off the membrane. Season the ribs with a dry rub.
2. Fire up the Pit Boss Wood Pellet Grill to 180 degrees F.
3. Place the ribs on the grill grate and smoke them for 4 hours.
4. Remove the ribs from the grill and increase the grill temperature to 350 degrees F.
5. Pour the BBQ sauce on a double-wall aluminium foil and place the ribs on top. Wrap the foil tightly.
6. Grill the wrapped ribs for 45 minutes.
7. Let the ribs rest for 20 minutes then slice.
8. Serve and enjoy.

Serving suggestion: Serve pork ribs with a fresh salad of choice

Variation Tip: use homemade rub and some apple cider vinegar

Nutrition-Per Serving:
Calories 220 | Fat 12g |Sodium 497 mg | Carbs 11g | Fiber 0.5g | Sugar 5g | Protein 3g

Roasted Pork Tenderloin

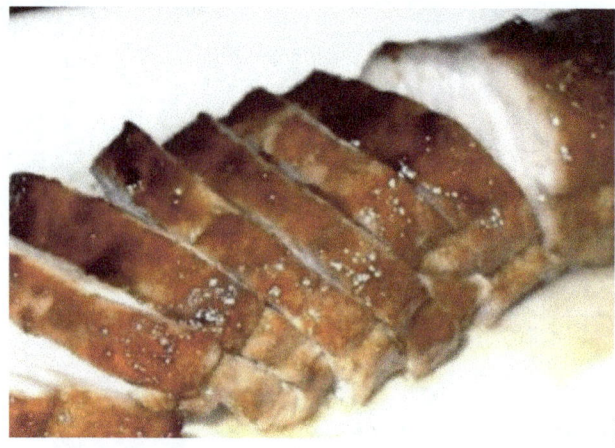

Prep Time: 15 minutes
Cook Time: 25 minutes
Serves: 4

Ingredients:

- 2 Pounds pork tenderloin
- Salt and black pepper to taste
- 2 tablespoons dried rosemary
- 2 tablespoons oil
- 1 lemon, sliced
- Basil for garnishing

Preparation:

1. Preheat the Pit Boss Wood Pellet Grill to 350 degrees F.
2. Rinse the pork and dry it with a paper towel then season it with salt, pepper, and rosemary.
3. Heat oil in a skillet and sear the pork for 2 minutes on each side.
4. Place the skillet on the grill grate and cook for 20 minutes.
5. Let the pork rest for 5 minutes then slice.
6. Serve the pork with lemon slices and garnish with basil.

Serving suggestion: Serve pork tenderloin with balsamic strawberry sauce

Variation Tip: Add strawberries to the skillet and roast them alongside the pork tenderloin

Nutrition-Per Serving:

Calories 360 | Fat 11g |Sodium 130 mg | Carbs 1g | Fiber 0.6g | Sugar 0g | Protein 60g

Grilled Crown Roast of Pork

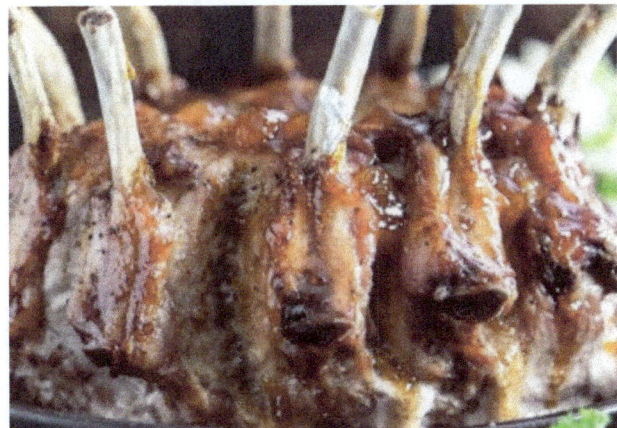

Prep Time: 5 minutes
Cook Time: 1 hour 30 minutes
Serves: 4

Ingredients:

- 1 crown roast of pork
- ¼ cup pork rub
- 1 cup apple juice
- 1 cup BBQ sauce

Preparation:

1. Fire up your Pit Boss Wood Pellet Grill to 375 degrees F.
2. Season the pork with pork rub and marinate for 30 minutes.
3. Wrap the tip of the crown roast of pork with aluminium foil and place them on the grill grate.
4. Grill the pork for 1 hour 30 minutes spraying the roast with apple juice after every 30 minutes during cooking.
5. Baste the crown roast of pork with BBQ sauce and allow the glaze to set.
6. Let the crown roast of pork rest for 15 minutes then slice.
7. Serve and enjoy.

Serving suggestion: Serve crown roast of pork ribs with a dipping sauce and some fresh salad

Variation Tip: use apple cider vinegar in place of apple juice or fresh or dried herbs for seasoning

Nutrition-Per Serving:
Calories 454 | Fat 19g | Sodium 1023 mg | Carbs 11g | Fiber 2g | Sugar 1g | Protein 57g

Grilled Wet-Rubbed Pork Ribs

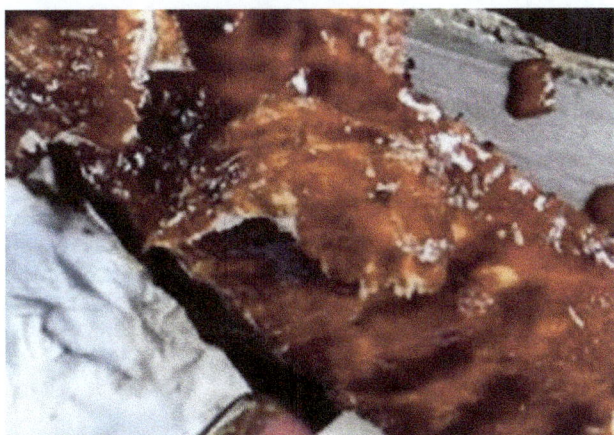

Prep Time: 15 minutes
Cook Time: 4 hours
Serves: 4

Ingredients:

- ½ cup brown sugar
- 1 tablespoon ground cumin
- 1 tablespoon ancho Chile powder
- 1 tablespoon smoked paprika
- 1 tablespoon garlic salt
- 3 tablespoons balsamic vinegar
- 1 rack pork ribs
- 2 cups apple juice

Preparation:

1. In a bowl mix sugar, cumin, ancho Chile powder, paprika, salt, and balsamic vinegar.
2. Season the pork with the wet rub and let it stand for 10 minutes.
3. Fire up your Pit Boss Wood Pellet Grill to 180 degrees F.
4. Place the ribs on the grill grate and smoke for 2 hours.
5. Transfer the ribs to a tin foil and raise the grill temperature to 250 degrees F.
6. Pour the apple juice into the tin foil and cook the ribs for 2 hours.
7. Let the ribs rest for 10 minutes then serve.

Serving suggestion: Serve wet-rubbed pork ribs with dipping sauce

Variation Tip: use apple cider vinegar in place of apple juice

Nutrition-Per Serving:

Calories 256 | Fat 4g | Sodium 1054 mg | Carbs 46g | Fiber 3g | Sugar 41g | Protein 30g

Grilled Cocoa-Crusted Pork Tenderloin

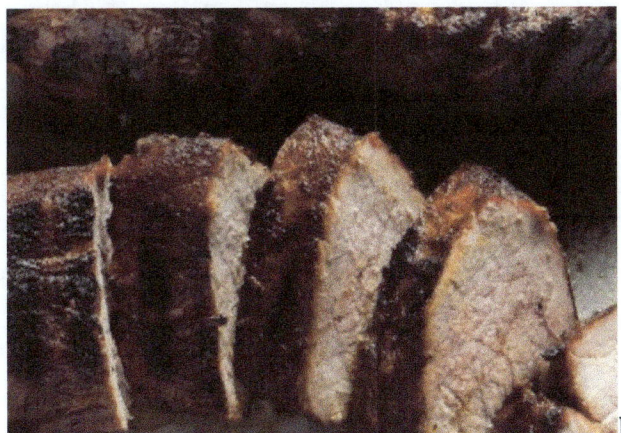

Prep Time: 40 minutes
Cook Time: 25 minutes
Serves: 2

Ingredients:

- 1 pork tenderloin
- ½ tablespoons ground fennel
- 2 tablespoons unsweetened cocoa powder
- 1 tablespoon smoked paprika
- ½ tablespoons salt
- ½ tablespoons black pepper
- 1 tablespoon oil
- 3 green onions, thinly sliced
- Dill for garnishing

Preparation:

1. Remove the connective tissue from the tenderloin.
2. Mix the remaining ingredients in a bowl and rub the tenderloin with the paste. Refrigerate the pork for 30 minutes.
3. Fire up the Pit Boss Wood Pellet Grill to 500 degrees F.
4. Sear the pork on the grill for about 3 minutes on each side.
5. Reduce the grill temperature to 350 degrees F and cook the pork for 15 minutes.
6. Remove the pork tenderloin from the grill and let it stand for 10 minutes before slicing.
7. Garnish the pork with dill and serve.

Serving suggestion: Serve pork tenderloin with grilled squash cubes

Variation Tip: process fennel seeds in the food processor and grill squash cubes sprinkled with oil alongside the pork

Nutrition-Per Serving:

Calories 382 | Fat 12g |Sodium 2152 mg | Carbs 7g | Fiber 5g | Sugar 1g | Protein 61g

Grilled Bone-in Pork Chops

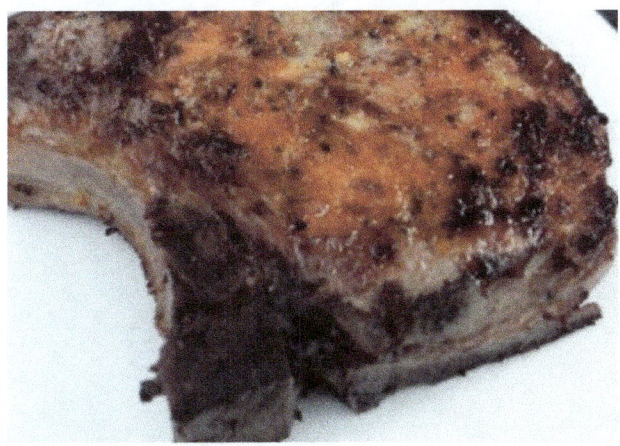

Prep Time: 5 minutes
Cook Time: 15 minutes
Serves: 6

Ingredients:

- 3 Pounds pork, cut into 6 chops
- ¼ cup BBQ rub
- Rosemary for garnishing

Preparation:

1. Fire up the Pit Boss Wood Pellet Grill to 450 degrees F.
2. Season the pork chops with the BBQ rub and place them on the grill grate.
3. Cook the pork chops for 6 minutes on each side.
4. Let the pork chops stand for 10 minutes.
5. Garnish the pork chops with rosemary then serve.

Serving suggestion: Serve pork chops with sautéed asparagus and sauce

Variation Tip: use some fresh herbs

Nutrition-Per Serving:
Calories 398 | Fat 19g |Sodium 363 mg | Carbs 8g | Fiber 1g | Sugar 6g | Protein 46g

LAMB RECIPES

Pit Boss Wood Pellet Grilled Lamb Chops

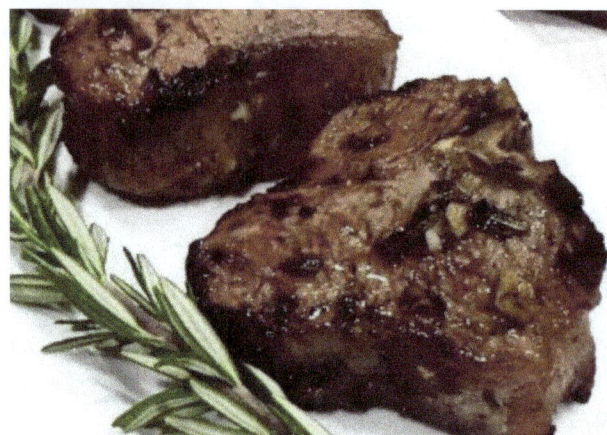

Prep Time: 1hour
Cook Time: 26 minutes
Serves: 3

Ingredients:

- 2 garlic cloves, crushed
- 1 tablespoon rosemary, freshly chopped
- 2 tablespoons oil
- 1 tablespoon lemon juice
- 1 tablespoon thyme leaves
- 1 tablespoon salt
- 9 lamb chops

Preparation:

1. Add garlic, rosemary, oil, lemon juice, thyme, and salt to a blender. Blend until smooth to make a marinade.
2. Rub the marinade on the chops then let marinate for 3 hours in the fridge.
3. Remove from the fridge and let sit at room temperature for 20 minutes.
4. Heat the Pit Boss Wood Pellet Grill to high heat until almost smoking. Sear the chops for 3 minutes per side.
5. Serve the chops with a green salad.

Serving suggestion: Serve lamb chops with corn and sautéed vegetables

Variation Tip: add garam masala, allspice, and cinnamon

Nutrition-Per Serving:
Calories 519 | Fat 44g |Sodium 861 mg | Carbs 2g | Fiber 0.3g | Sugar 0.7g | Protein 24g

Grilled Leg of Lamb Roast with Carrots

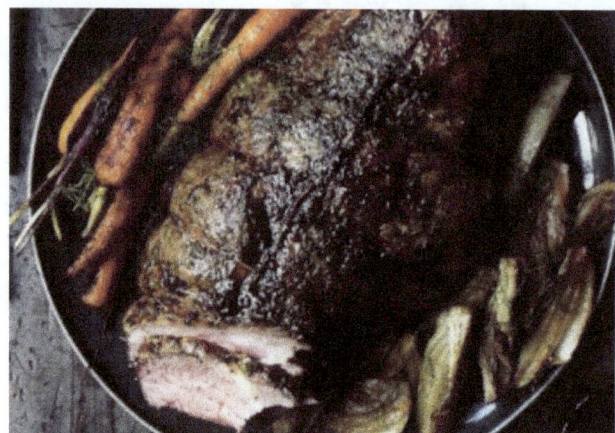

Prep Time: 30 minutes
Cook Time: 2 hours
Serves: 8

Ingredients:

- 5 Pounds leg of lamb roast, boneless

For the Rub
- 1 tablespoon raw sugar
- 1 tablespoon salt
- 1 tablespoon black pepper
- 1 tablespoon smoked paprika
- 1 tablespoon garlic powder
- 1 tablespoon rosemary
- 1 tablespoon onion powder
- 1 tablespoon cumin
- ½ tablespoons cayenne pepper

For the carrots
- 1 bunch carrots
- oil
- Salt and pepper to taste

Preparation:

1. Preheat your Pit Boss Wood Pellet Grill to 375 degrees F.
2. Meanwhile, trim fat from the roast such that it's not more than ¼ inch thick.
3. In a mixing bowl, combine all the rub ingredients and generously rub the mixture all over the lamb roast.
4. Place the lamb in the grill and set to smoke for 2 hours.

5. Toss carrots in oil, salt, and pepper then add them at 1½ hour. Check if the internal temperature of the lamb is 90 degrees F.
6. Cook for the remaining time or until the internal temperature reaches 135 degrees F.
7. Remove the lamb roast from the grill and let rest for 15 minutes while covered with foil.
8. Remove the carrots from the grill and serve with the lamb. Enjoy.

Serving suggestion: Serve lamb roast with sautéed broccoli and homemade sauce of choice

Variation Tip: grill with other vegetables such as potatoes

Nutrition-Per Serving:
Calories 256 | Fat 8g |Sodium 431 mg | Carbs 6g | Fiber 1g | Sugar 3g | Protein 36g

Grilled Lamb with Sugar Glaze

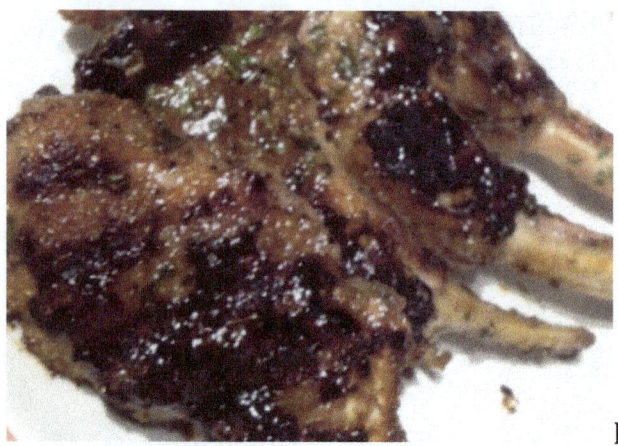

Prep Time: 1hour 15 minutes
Cook Time: 10 minutes
Serves: 4

Ingredients:

- ¼ cup brown sugar
- 2 tablespoons ginger, ground
- 2 tablespoons tarragon, dried
- 1 tablespoon cinnamon, ground
- 1 tablespoon garlic powder
- ½ tablespoons salt
- 1 tablespoon black pepper
- 4 lamb chops

Preparation:

1. In a mixing bowl, mix sugar, ginger, tarragon, cinnamon, garlic powder, salt, and pepper to make a rub.
2. Rub the seasoning on the lamb chops then place on a plate, cover, and refrigerate for 1 hour.
3. Fire up your grill to high heat and brush the grill grate with oil.
4. Grill for 5 minutes on each side. Remove the chops from the grill and let cool before serving.

Serving suggestion: Serve the lamb with cooked green peas and potato wedges

Variation Tip: use an herb blend of parsley, chives, and tarragon in place of dried tarragon

Nutrition-Per Serving:
Calories 241 | Fat 13g |Sodium 339 mg | Carbs 16g | Fiber 1g | Sugar 14g | Protein 15g

Grilled Leg of Lamb

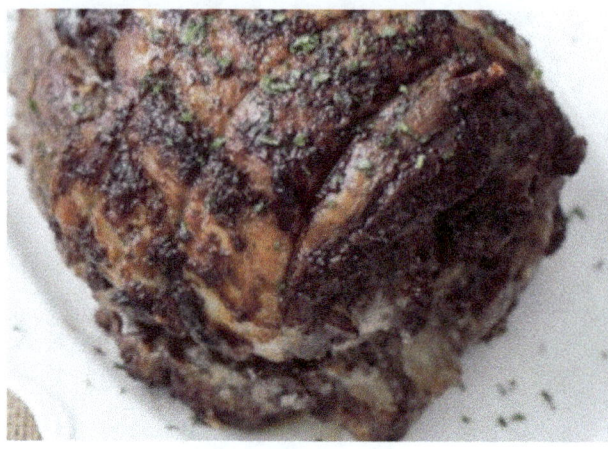

Prep Time: 10 minutes
Cook Time: 10 minutes
Serves: 4

Ingredients:

- 4 lamb steaks
- ¼ cup oil
- 4 cloves garlic, minced
- 1 tablespoon rosemary, freshly chopped
- Salt and pepper to taste

Preparation:

1. Place lamb steaks in a shallow dish then cover with oil, garlic, rosemary, salt, and pepper.
2. Coat the steak on all sides with the rub then let sit for 30 minutes.
3. Fire up the Pit Boss Wood Pellet Grill to high heat then lightly oil the grill grates.
4. Cook the steak for 5 minutes on each side or until it has an internal temperature of 140 degrees F

Serving suggestion: Serve the leg of lamb with sauteed broccoli and carrots

Variation Tip: use roasted garlic powder in place of minced garlic

Nutrition-Per Serving:
Calories 327 | Fat 22g | Sodium 112 mg | Carbs 2g | Fiber 0.2g | Sugar 0.2g | Protein 30g

Grilled Spicy Lamb Skewers

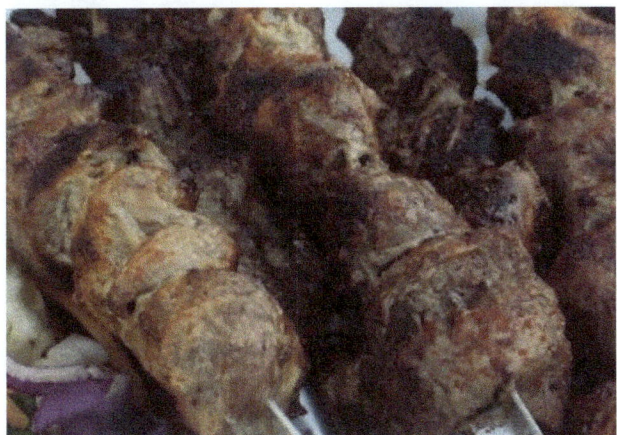

Prep Time: 20 minutes
Cook Time: 6 minutes
Serves: 10

Ingredients:

- 1 Pound lamb shoulder, cut into cubes
- 10 skewers
- 2 tablespoons cumin, ground
- 2 tablespoons red pepper flakes
- 1 tablespoon salt

Preparation:

1. Thread all the lamb cubes on skewers.
2. Preheat your Pit Boss Wood Pellet Grill to medium heat then lightly grease the grill grates with oil.
3. Place the skewers on the grill grates and cook while turning as you sprinkle cumin, salt, and red pepper flakes.
4. Cook for 6 minutes or until the meat is well browned. Serve and enjoy.

Serving suggestion: Serve skewers with garlic butter sauce

Variation Tip: Add vegetables to the skewers

Nutrition-Per Serving:
Calories 77 | Fat 5g | Sodium 714 mg | Carbs 2g | Fiber 0.6g | Sugar 0.2g | Protein 6g

Smoked Lamb Chops

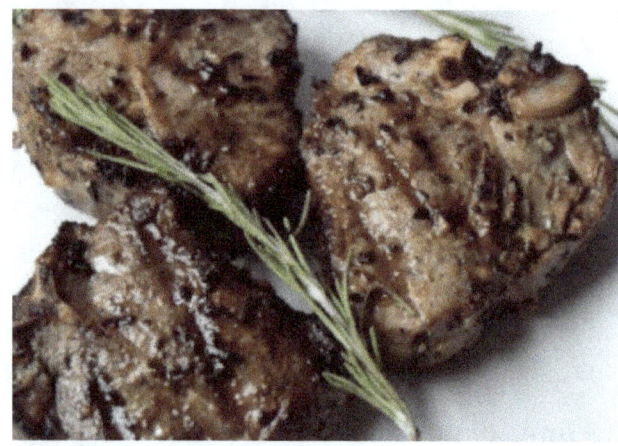

Prep Time: 10 minutes
Cook Time: 50 minutes
Serves: 4

Ingredients:

- 1 rack of lamb
- ¼ cup oil
- 2 tablespoons freshly ground rosemary
- 2 tablespoons freshly ground sage
- 2 tablespoons shallots, roughly chopped
- 1 tablespoon freshly ground thyme
- 2 minced garlic cloves
- ½ tablespoons salt
- ½ tablespoons black pepper
- 1 tablespoon honey
- Basil for garnishing

Preparation:

1. Remove the silver skin from the rack of lamb and trim off excess fat.
2. Mix the remaining ingredients in a bowl and apply the paste to the lamb.
3. Place the lamb in a plastic wrapper and refrigerate for 24 hours.
4. Remove the lamb from the refrigerator 1 hour before cooking.
5. Fire up your Pit Boss Wood Pellet Grill to 180 degrees F.
6. Place the lamb on the grill and smoke for 1 hour.
7. Remove the lamb from the grill grate and increase the grill temperature to 500 degrees F. Sear the lamb for 2 minutes on each side.
8. Let the rack of lamb rest for 10 minutes then slice into chops.
9. Garnish the lamb with basil and serve.

Serving suggestion: Serve lamb chops with root vegetable puree

Variation Tip: use the combination of your favourite herbs

Nutrition-Per Serving:
Calories 613 | Fat 56g |Sodium 362 mg | Carbs 7g | Fiber 1g | Sugar 5g | Protein 19g

Smoked Lamb Shoulder

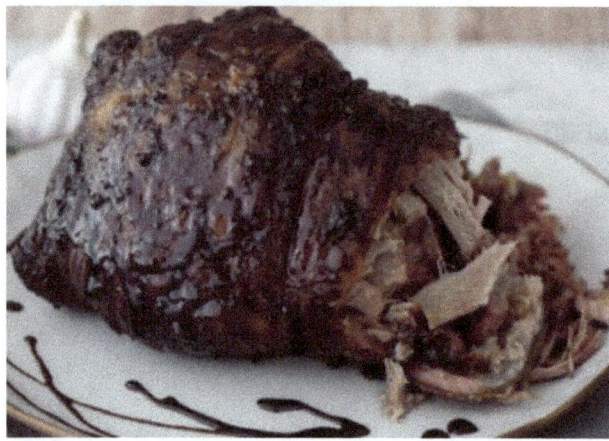

Prep Time: 15 minutes
Cook Time: 6 hours
Serves: 6

Ingredients:

- 5 Pounds lamb shoulder
- 2 tablespoons oil
- ¼ cup ultimate dry rub
- ½ cup apple cider vinegar
- ½ cup apple juice
- Rosemary for garnishing

Preparation:

1. Fire up your Pit Boss Wood Pellet Grill to 225 degrees F.
2. Trim off excess fat and cartilage from the lamb shoulder.
3. Mix oil and dry rub in a bowl then coat both sides of the lamb with the paste.
4. Place the lamb shoulders on a flat surface and roll it. Tie the shoulder with butcher twine.
5. Place the lamb on the grill and smoke for 3 hours.
6. Spritz the lamb shoulder with apple cider vinegar and apple juice.
7. Cook the lamb for an additional 3 hours, spraying it after every 1 hour of cooking.
8. Remove the lamb from the grill and let it rest for 30 minutes.
9. Garnish the lamb with rosemary and serve.

Serving suggestion: Pull the lamb and serve it in pita bread with tzatziki sauce

Variation Tip: use the combination of your favourite herbs

Nutrition-Per Serving:
Calories 378 | Fat 17g |Sodium 167 mg | Carbs 4g | Fiber 1g | Sugar 2g | Protein 47g

Smoked Lamb Meatballs

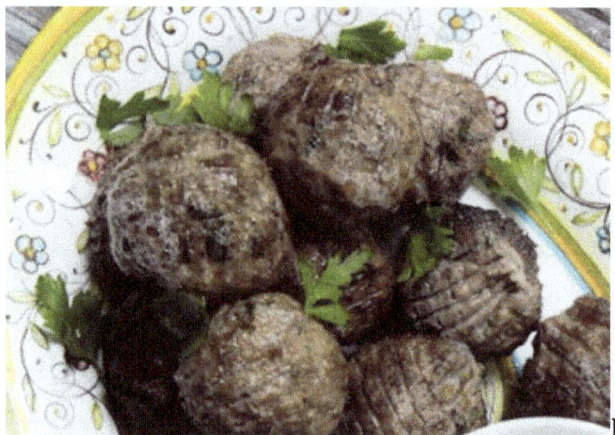

Prep Time: 10 minutes
Cook Time: 1 hour
Serves: 4

Ingredients:

- 1 Pound lamb shoulder, ground
- ¼ cup panko breadcrumbs
- 3 tablespoons diced shallot
- 3 garlic cloves, finely diced
- 1 egg
- 1 tablespoon salt
- ½ tablespoons black pepper
- ½ tablespoons cumin
- ½ tablespoons smoked paprika
- ¼ tablespoons red pepper flakes
- ¼ tablespoons ground cinnamon

Preparation:

1. Fire up your Pit Boss Wood Pellet Grill to 250 degrees F.
2. In a bowl mix all the ingredients until well combined.
3. Scoop 1 spoonful of the lamb mixture and knead into the form of balls. Place the meatballs on a baking sheet.
4. Place the baking sheet on the grill and cook for 1 hour.
5. Remove the meatballs from the grill and serve immediately.

Serving suggestion: Serve the meatballs with lettuce and sauce in pita bread or alongside pasta

Variation Tip: use the combination of your favourite coriander

Nutrition-Per Serving:
Calories 385 | Fat 20g | Sodium 1660 mg | Carbs 4g | Fiber 1g | Sugar 1g | Protein 37g

Grilled Crown Rack of Lamb

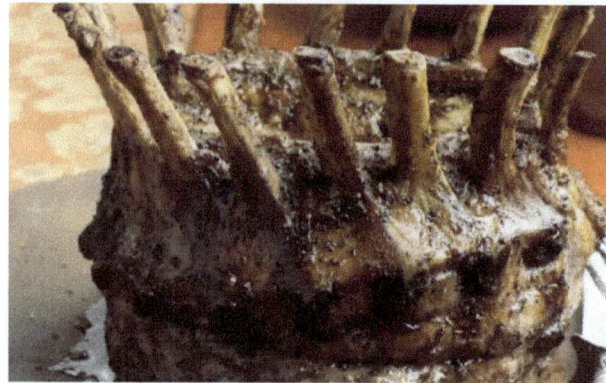

Prep Time: 10 minutes
Cook Time: 30 minutes
Serves: 6

Ingredients:

- 2 racks of lamb, drenched
- 1 tablespoon minced garlic cloves
- 1 tablespoon finely chopped rosemary
- ½ cup oil

Preparation:

1. Rinse the rack of lamb with cold water and dry them with a paper towel.
2. Make a ¼-inch cut down between each bone.
3. Mix the remaining ingredients in a bowl and brush the lamb with the paste.
4. Bend each rack of lamb into a semicircle then put them together to form a circle.
5. Tie the rack of lamb tightly with a butcher's twine to form a crown shape.
6. Fire up your Pit Boss Wood Pellet Grill to 450 degrees F.
7. Place the crown rack of lamb on a baking sheet and cook for 10 minutes.
8. Reduce the grill temperature to 300 degrees F and cook for 20 minutes.
9. Remove the rack of lamb from the grill and let it rest for 15 minutes.
10. Serve the lamb while hot.

Serving suggestion: serve the crown rack of lamb with roasted potatoes or veggies

Variation Tip: Use coriander, vinegar, Dijon mustard, and thyme

Nutrition-Per Serving:
Calories 645 | Fat 44g | Sodium 1511 mg | Carbs 1g | Fiber 0.5g | Sugar 0g | Protein 63g

Smoked Leg of Lamb

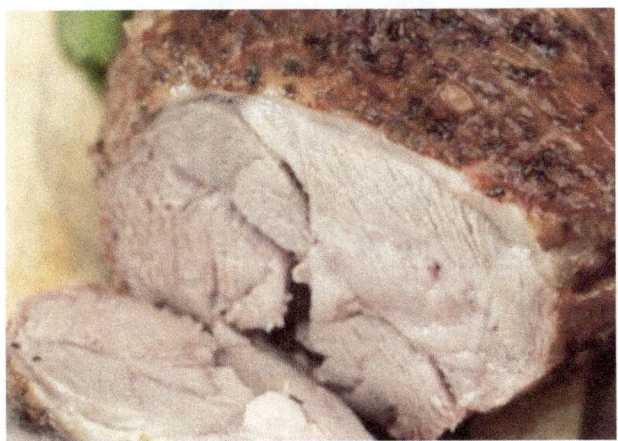

Prep Time: 15 minutes
Cook Time: 4 hours
Serves: 6

Ingredients
- 2 Pounds leg of lamb
- 4 minced garlic cloves
- 2 tablespoons salt
- 1 tablespoon black pepper
- 2 tablespoons oregano
- 1 tablespoon thyme
- 2 tablespoons oil
- Rosemary

Preparation:
1. Clean the leg of the lamb
2. Trim off excess fat from the leg of lamb.
3. Mix the remaining ingredients in a bowl and rub the paste over the lamb.
4. Wrap the lamb with a plastic wrapper and marinate for 1 hour.
5. Fire up your Pit Boss Wood Pellet Grill to 250 degrees F.
6. Place the lamb on the grill and cook it for 4 hours.
7. Remove the leg from the grill and slice.
8. Garnish the lamb with rosemary and serve.

Serving suggestion: serve the leg of lamb with sauteed zucchini and squash

Variation Tip: Use fresh herbs and lemon juice

Nutrition-Per Serving:
Calories 356 | Fat 16g | Sodium 2474 mg | Carbs 3g | Fiber 1g | Sugar 1g | Protein 49g

CHICKEN RECIPES

Grilled Buffalo Chicken legs

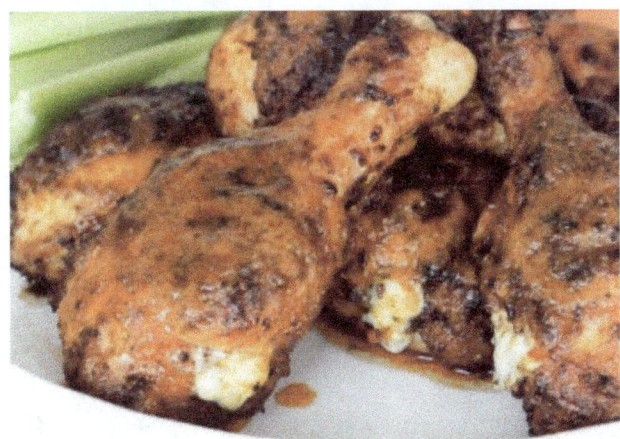

Prep Time: 5 minutes
Cook Time: 50 minutes
Serves: 6

Ingredients:

- 12 chicken legs
- 1 tablespoon Buffalo seasoning
- ½ tablespoons salt
- 1 cup Buffalo sauce

Preparation:

1. Fire up your Pit Boss Wood Pellet Grill 325 degrees F.
2. Toss the chicken legs with seasoning and salt then place them in the grill.
3. Grill for 40 minutes while turning occasionally during the cooking period.
4. Brush the legs chicken with buffalo sauce and cook for an additional 10 minutes or until the internal temperature reaches 165 degrees F.
5. Remove the chicken wings from the grill, brush with more sauce and serve.

Serving suggestion: serve chicken leg with celery stalks and ranch

Variation Tip: add mayo, garlic, and spicy chorizo

Nutrition-Per Serving:
Calories 956 | Fat 47g |Sodium 1750 mg | Carbs 1g | Fiber 0g | Sugar 0g | Protein 124g

Grilled Chile lime chicken Breast

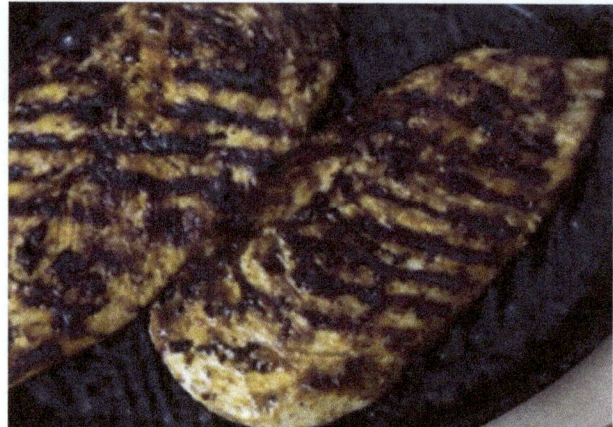

Prep Time: 5 minutes
Cook Time: 15 minutes
Serves: 1

Ingredients:

- 1 chicken breast
- 1 tablespoon oil
- ½ tablespoons Chile-lime seasoning
- Salt to taste

Preparation:

1. Fire up your Pit Boss Wood Pellet to 400 degrees F.
2. Lightly coat the chicken breast with oil then sprinkle with lime seasoning and salt.
3. Place the chicken breast in the preheated grill and cook for 6 minutes per side or until the internal temperature reaches 165 degrees F.
4. Serve and enjoy.

Serving suggestion: serve the chicken breast on salad and rice

Variation Tip: use grated lime peel, lime juice, and jalapeno Chile in place of Chile-lime seasoning

Nutrition-Per Serving:
Calories 131 | Fat 5g |Sodium 235 mg | Carbs 4g | Fiber 1g | Sugar 1g | Protein 19g

Grilled Chicken Flatbread

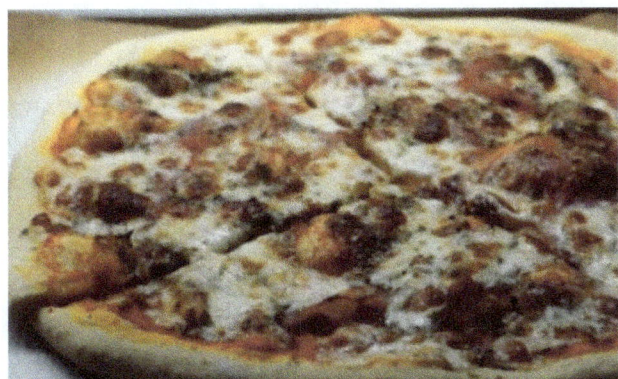

Prep Time: 5 minutes
Cook Time: 30 minutes
Serves: 6

Ingredients:

- 6 pita bread, mini
- 1½ cups buffalo sauce
- 4 cups chicken breasts, cooked and cubed
- 3 cups mozzarella cheese
- Blue cheese for drizzling

Preparation:

1. Preheat your Pit Boss Wood Pellet Grill to 400 degrees F.
2. Meanwhile, place the pita breads on a working surface and spread buffalo sauce on each.
3. Toss the chicken breast cubes in buffalo sauce then divide them among the 6 breads.
4. Top each bread with cheese then place them on the grill grates and over indirect heat.
5. Close the lid and cook for 7 minutes or until the cheese has melted.
6. Remove the mini pizzas from the grill and drizzle with blue cheese. Serve.

Serving suggestion: serve with blue cheese and ranch

Variation Tip: use Cholula buffalo sauce

Nutrition-Per Serving:
Calories 311 | Fat 25g |Sodium 235 mg | Carbs 7g | Fiber 1g | Sugar 1g | Protein 29g

Grilled Miso Chicken wings

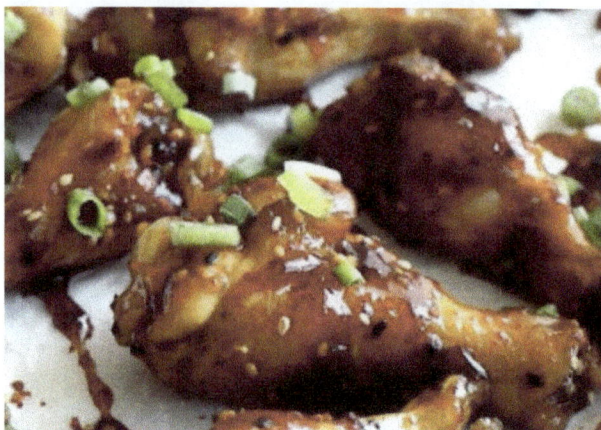

Prep Time: 20 minutes
Cook Time: 45 minutes
Serves: 6

Ingredients:

- ¾ cup soy
- ½ cup pineapple juice
- 1 tablespoon sriracha
- ⅛ cup miso
- ⅛ cup gochujang
- ½ cup water
- ½ cup oil
- 2 Pounds chicken wings
- Togarashi

Preparation:

1. Combine all ingredients in a mixing bowl. Toss the chicken wings with the marinade until well coated.
2. Let marinate in the fridge for 12 hours.
3. Preheat your Pit Boss Wood Pellet Grill to 375 degrees F.
4. Place the chicken wings on the grill grates and close the lid. Cook for 45 minutes or until the internal temperature reaches 165 degrees F.
5. Remove the chicken wings from the grill and sprinkle with togarashi. Serve.

Serving suggestion: Serve the chicken wings with grilled vegetable pasta salad

Variation Tip: add dark brown sugar and sake

Nutrition-Per Serving:

Calories 703 | Fat 56g |Sodium 1156 mg | Carbs 24g | Fiber 1g | Sugar 6g | Protein 27g

Grilled BBQ Chicken Wings

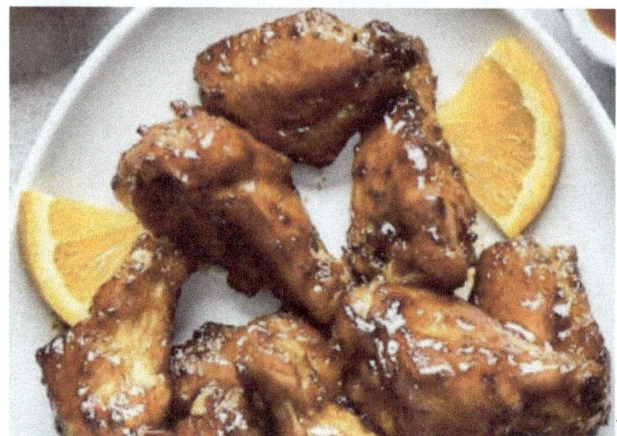

Prep Time: 10 minutes
Cook Time: 30 minutes
Serves: 4

Ingredients:

- 1½ Pounds chicken wings
- Salt and pepper to taste
- Garlic powder
- Onion powder
- Cayenne
- Paprika
- Seasoning salt
- BBQ sauce

Preparation:

1. Preheat your Pit Boss Wood Pellet Grill to low heat.
2. Mix all the seasoning in a mixing bowl to make a rub then generously season the chicken wings with it.
3. Grill the chicken wings for 20 minutes while turning them occasionally.
4. Remove the wings from the grill and let them cool for 5 minutes.
5. Toss them with BBQ sauce and serve with a salad of choice.

Serving suggestion: serve the BBQ Chicken wings cheesy orzo

Variation Tip: Use homemade BBQ sauce

Nutrition-Per Serving:
Calories 311 | Fat 15g | Sodium 1400 mg | Carbs 22g | Fiber 3g | Sugar 12g | Protein 22g

Grilled Buffalo Chicken Breast

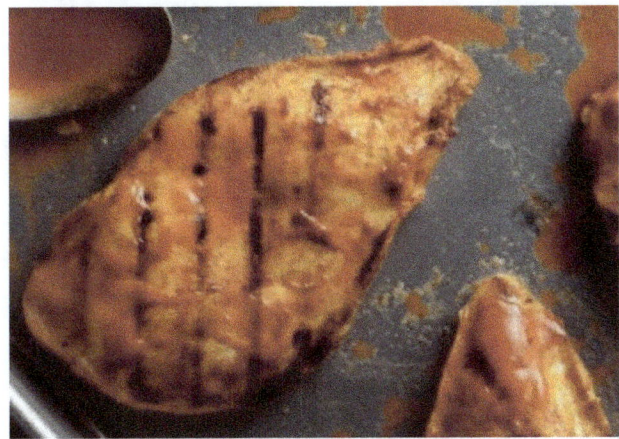

Prep Time: 10 minutes
Cook Time: 25 minutes
Serves: 6

Ingredients:

- 5 chicken breasts, boneless
- 2 tablespoons BBQ rub
- 1 cup buffalo sauce

Preparation:

1. Preheat your Pit Boss Wood Pellet Grill to 400 degrees F.
2. Meanwhile, slice the chicken breasts into long strips then rub the BBQ rub.
3. Place the chicken breast strips in your gill then paint both sides with BBQ sauce.
4. Grill for 4 minutes, flip, and paint with BBQ sauce. Continues with the princess until the internal temperature reaches 165 degrees F.
5. Remove from the grill, let cool, and serve.

Serving suggestion: serve Buffalo chicken breast with pan-fried potato wedges or salad

Variation Tip: Use homemade Cholula sauce or green jalapeno sauce in place of buffalo sauce

Nutrition-Per Serving:
Calories 176 | Fat 4g | Sodium 631 mg | Carbs 1g | Fiber 0g | Sugar 1g | Protein 32g

Grilled Chicken Kabobs

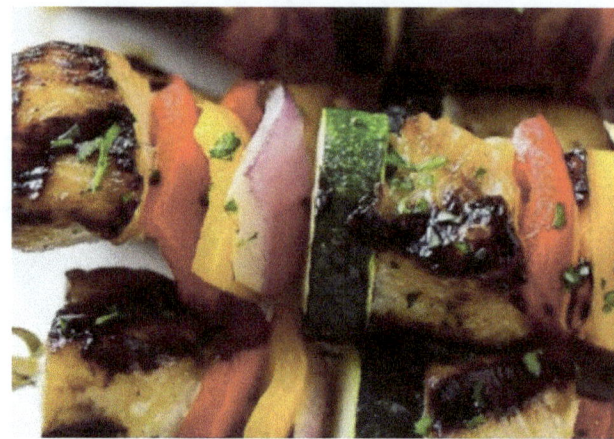

Prep Time: 45 minutes
Cook Time: 12 minutes
Serves: 6

Ingredients:

- ½ cup oil
- 2 tablespoons white vinegar
- 1 tablespoon lemon juice
- 1½ tablespoons salt
- ½ tablespoons coarsely ground black pepper
- 2 tablespoons freshly chopped chives
- 1½ tablespoons freshly chopped thyme
- 2 tablespoons freshly chopped parsley
- 1 tablespoon minced garlic
- 2 chopped bell peppers (red and yellow)
- 1½ Pounds chicken breast, boneless and skinless, cut into small chops
- Parsley for topping

Preparation:

1. In a bowl mix oil, white vinegar, lemon juice, salt, black pepper, chives, thyme, parsley, and garlic.
2. Add the bell pepper and chicken to the marinade and toss to mix. Marinate for 30 minutes.
3. Preheat the Pit Boss Wood Pellet Grill to 450 degrees F.
4. Assemble the kabobs and place them on the grill.
5. Cook the kabobs for 12 minutes flipping them halfway through cooking.
6. Top the kabobs with parsley and serve.

Serving suggestion: serve the chicken kabobs with Caesar dressing

Variation Tip: experiment with different vegetables

Nutrition-Per Serving:

Calories 165| Fat 9g |Sodium 582 mg | Carbs 2g | Fiber 0.3 g | Sugar 0.4 g | Protein 23g

Grilled Whole Chicken

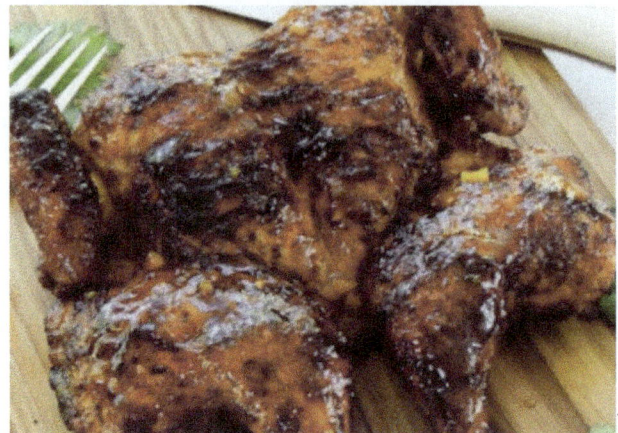

Prep Time: 10 minutes
Cook Time: 1 hour 10 minutes
Serves: 6

Ingredients:

- 5 Pounds whole chicken
- ½ cup oil
- ½ cup chicken rub
- Topping: sliced lemon and rosemary

Preparation:

1. Preheat your Pit Boss Wood Pellet Grill to 450 degrees F.
2. Tie the chicken legs together with a butcher's twine.
3. Brush the chicken with oil then coat it with chicken rub.
4. Grill the chicken for 1 hour and 10 minutes.
5. Remove the chicken from the grill and let it rest for 15 minutes
6. Top the chicken with lemon slices and rosemary.
7. Serve and enjoy.

Serving suggestion: serve the chicken with baked potato salad.

Variation Tip: a homemade chicken seasoning can be used in place of chicken rub.

Nutrition-Per Serving:
Calories 935| Fat 53g |Sodium 320 mg | Carbs 1g | Fiber 0 g | Sugar 0 g | Protein 107g

Grilled Chicken Breast

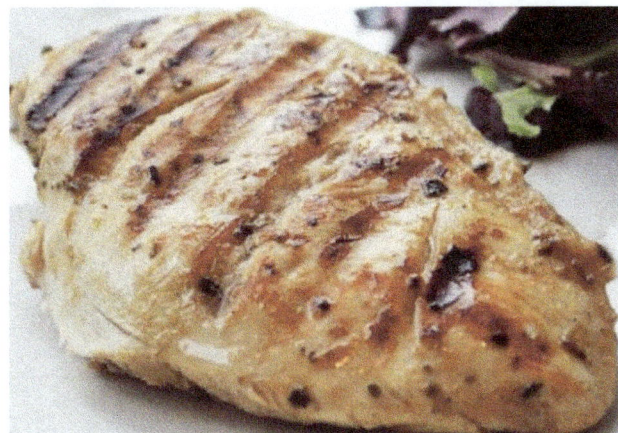

Prep Time: 10 minutes
Cook Time: 15 minutes
Serves: 6

Ingredients:

- 3 chicken breasts
- 1 tablespoon oil
- ¾ tablespoons salt
- ¼ tablespoons garlic powder
- ¼ tablespoons onion powder
- Topping: lemon wedges and rosemary

Preparation:

1. Fire up your Pit Boss Wood Pellet Grill to 375 degrees F.
2. Coat the chicken with oil then season with salt, garlic powder, and onion powder.
3. Place the chicken on the grill grate and cook for 7 minutes on each side.
4. Top the chicken with lemon with rosemary then serve.

Serving suggestion: Serve the chicken breast with your favourite salad.

Variation Tip: balsamic vinegar can be mixed with seasonings to make a marinade.

Nutrition-Per Serving:
Calories 120| Fat 4g |Sodium 309 mg | Carbs 1g | Fiber 0 g | Sugar 0 g | Protein 19g

Pit Boss Wood Pellet Smoked Spatchcock Turkey

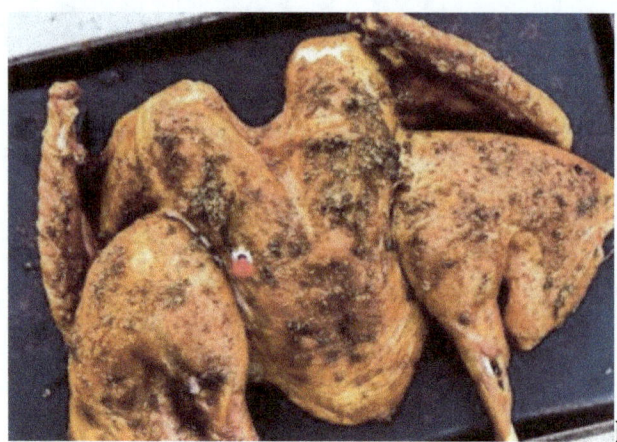

Prep Time: 30 minutes
Cook Time: 1 hour 15 minutes
Serves: 8

Ingredients:

- 1 whole turkey
- ½ cup oil
- ¼ cup chicken rub
- 1 tablespoon onion powder
- 1 tablespoon garlic powder
- 1 tablespoon rubbed sage

For Garnishing:

- Parsley
- 1 orange, sliced
- 1 lemon sliced

Preparation:

1. Fire up your Pit Boss Wood Pellet Grill to 500 degrees F.
2. Place the turkey on a flat surface with the breast side down.
3. Cut up both sides of the backbone through the ribs and remove the spine.
4. Rub both sides of the turkey with oil and season it with chicken rub, onion powder, garlic powder, and sage.
5. Place the turkey on the grill with the skin side up. Grill the turkey for 30 minutes.
6. Reduce the grill temperature to 325 degrees F and grill for an additional 45 minutes.
7. Remove the turkey from the grill and let it rest for 20 minutes.
8. Garnish the turkey with parsley, orange slices, and lemon slices.

9. Serve and enjoy.

Serving suggestion: serve the spatchcock turkey with mashed potatoes.

Variation Tip: preferred seasoning can be used.

Nutrition-Per Serving:
Calories 724| Fat 38g |Sodium 165 mg | Carbs 2g | Fiber 0 g | Sugar 0 g | Protein 89g

Smoked Cornish Hen

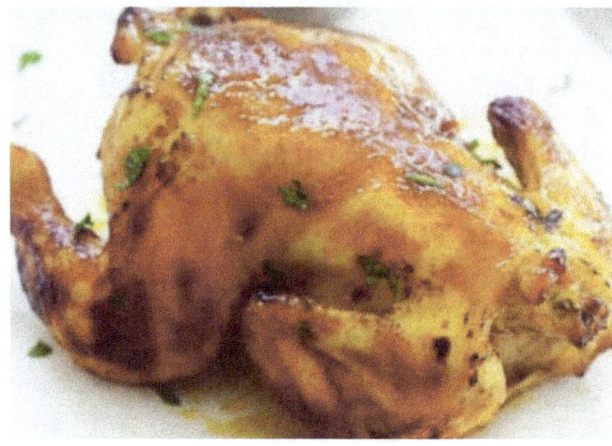

Prep Time: 10 minutes
Cook Time: 1 hour
Serves: 6

Ingredients:

- 6 cornish hens
- 2 tablespoons oil
- 6 tablespoons chicken rub

Preparation:

1. Fire up your Pit Boss Wood Pellet Grill to 275 degrees F.
2. Brush the hens with oil then coat them with chicken rub.
3. Place the hens on the grill with the breast side down and smoke for 30 minutes.
4. Remove the hens from the grill and raise the grill temperature to 400 degrees F.
5. Return the hens on the grill with the breast side up and cook for about 30 minutes until the internal temperature is 165 degrees F.
6. Let the hens rest for 10 minutes then serve.

Serving suggestion: serve the cornish hen with creamy noodles.

Variation Tip: seasoning of your choice can be used.

Nutrition-Per Serving:
Calories 696| Fat 50g |Sodium 165 mg | Carbs 1g | Fiber 0 g | Sugar 0 g | Protein 57g

Smoked Chicken Wings

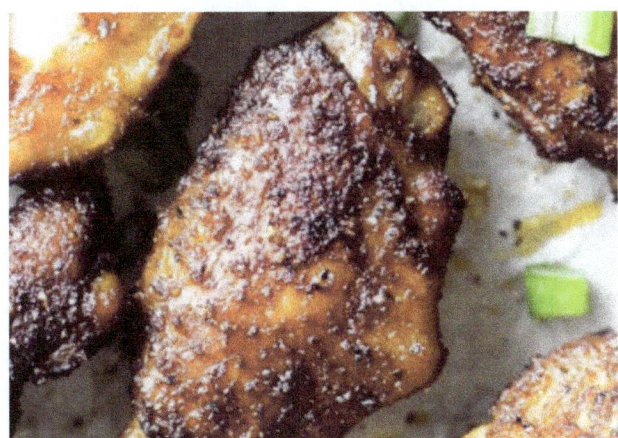

Prep Time: 10 minutes
Cook Time: 2 hours
Serves: 6

Ingredients:

- 3 lb chicken wings
- 1 tbsp all-purpose seasoning
- Buffalo sauce

Preparation:

1. Fire up your Pit Boss Wood Pellet Grill to 180 degrees F.
2. Coat the chicken wings with the all-purpose seasoning and place them on the grill.
3. Smoke the wings for 2 hours turning them halfway through the smoking process.
4. Remove the chicken wings from the grill and raise the grill temperature to 375 degrees F.
5. Place the wings back on the grill and cook for about 6 minutes.
6. Drain excess grease from the wings then toss them in buffalo sauce.
7. Serve and enjoy.

Serving suggestion: Serve the chicken wings with roasted broccoli.

Variation Tip: buffalo sauce can be replaced with a sauce of choice.

Nutrition-Per Serving:
Calories 755| Fat 55g |Sodium 1747 mg | Carbs 24g | Fiber 1 g | Sugar 2 g | Protein 39g

VEGAN AND VEGETARIAN RECIPES

Pit Boss Wood Pellet Grill-Smoked Asparagus

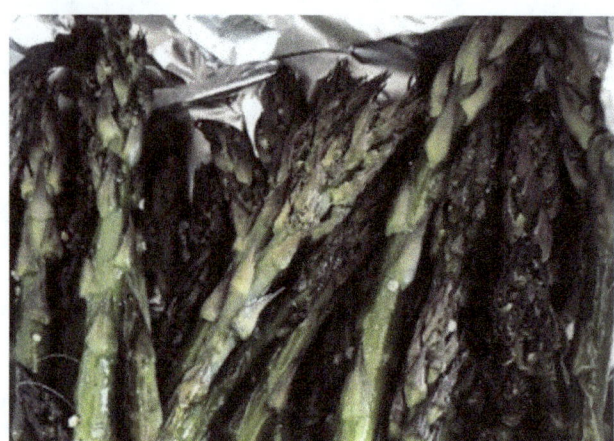

Prep Time: 10 minutes
Cook Time: 1hour
Serves: 4

Ingredients:

- 1 bunch asparagus
- 2 tablespoons oil
- Salt and pepper to taste

Preparation:

1. Set your Pit Boss Wood Pellet Grill to smoke.
2. Meanwhile, trim the asparagus ends and put them in a mixing bowl.
3. Drizzle oil then season them with salt and pepper.
4. Transfer them to tinfoil and fold the sides to create a basket.
5. Place the basket in the grill and smoke the asparagus for 1-hour or until they are soft.
6. Serve.

Serving suggestion: serve smoked asparagus with smoked turkey breast.

Variation Tip: use sliced garlic cloves and onions

Nutrition-Per Serving:
Calories 43| Fat 2g |Sodium 148 mg | Carbs 4g | Fiber 2 g | Sugar 2 g | Protein 3g

Baked Sweet Potatoes

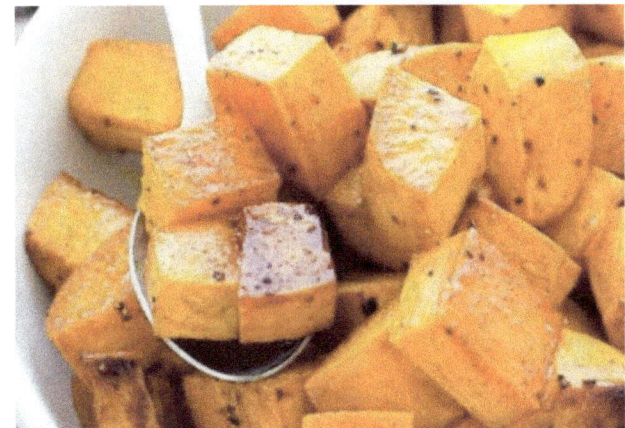

Prep Time: 10 minutes
Cook Time: 35 minutes
Serves: 4

Ingredients:

- 2 Pounds sweet potatoes
- 1 red onion, chopped
- 2 tablespoons oil
- 2 tablespoons orange juice
- 1 tablespoon roasted cinnamon
- 1 tablespoon salt
- ¼ tablespoons chipotle chili pepper

Preparation:

1. Preheat your Pit Boss Wood Pellet Grill to 425 degrees F.
2. Meanwhile, toss the sweet potatoes and onions in oil and orange juice.
3. In a separate bowl, mix salt and chili pepper then sprinkle the mixture over the potatoes. Toss until well coated.
4. Spread the sweet potatoes in a lined baking pan then place the pan in the grill.
5. Bake for 35 minutes or until the sweet potatoes are tender and golden brown.
6. Serve and enjoy.

Serving suggestion: serve roasted sweet potato with roasted pork.

Variation Tip: use yellow onion instead of red onion.

Nutrition-Per Serving:
Calories 145| Fat 5g |Sodium 428 mg | Carbs 23g | Fiber 4 g | Sugar 16 g | Protein 2g

Smoked Stuffed mushrooms

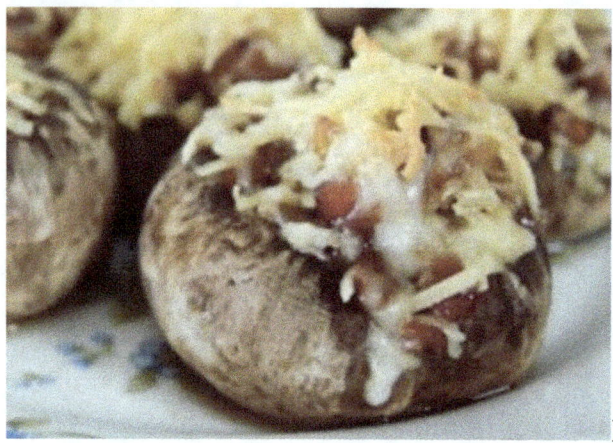

Prep Time: 10 minutes
Cook Time: 1 hour 20 minutes
Serves: 12

Ingredients:

- 12 white mushrooms
- ½ cup bread crumbs
- ½ cup parmesan cheese
- 2 garlic cloves, minced
- 2 tablespoons fresh parsley
- ⅓ cup oil
- Salt and pepper to taste

Preparation:

1. Preheat your Pit Boss Wood Pellet Grill to 180 degrees F.
2. Remove the stems from the mushrooms. Wash the stems and dice them into small pieces.
3. Mix the mushroom stems, bread crumbs, cheese, garlic, parsley, 3 tablespoons oil, salt, and pepper.
4. Arrange the mushrooms in a pan then fill them with the cheese mixture until they are heaping. Drizzle more oil.
5. Place the pan in the grill and smoke for 1 hour 20 minutes or until the mushrooms are tender.
6. Remove from the grill and serve.

Serving suggestion: serve the stuffed mushrooms with your favourite simple salad.

Variation Tip: Use mozzarella cheese in place of parmesan cheese.

Nutrition-Per Serving:

Calories 319| Fat 8g |Sodium 840 mg | Carbs 26g | Fiber 3 g | Sugar 14 g | Protein 17g

Grilled Stuffed Zucchini

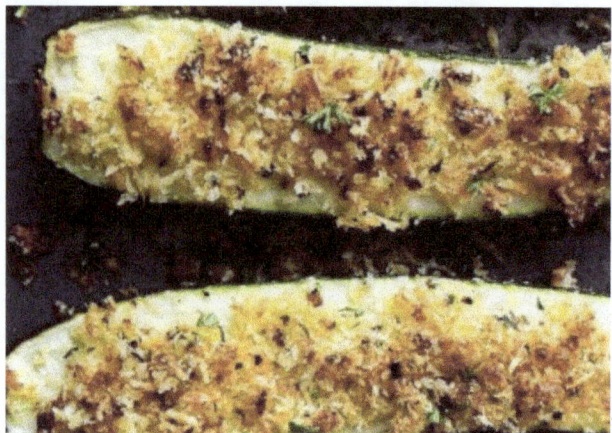

Prep Time: 10 minutes
Cook Time: 11 minutes
Serves: 4

Ingredients:

- 4 zucchinis
- 5 tablespoons oil
- 2 tablespoons red onion
- ¼ garlic cloves, minced
- ½ cup bread crumbs
- ½ cup mozzarella cheese, shredded
- 1 tablespoon fresh mint
- ½ tablespoons salt
- 3 tablespoons parmesan cheese

Preparation:

1. Cut the zucchini lengthwise and scoop out the pulp.
2. Brush the shells with 2 tablespoons oil.
3. Sauté pulp and onions in the remaining oil in a pan. Add garlic and cook for an additional 1 minute. Add crumbs and cook for 2 minutes or until golden brown.
4. Remove from heat and stir in cheese, mint, and salt. Spoon the mixture into the zucchini halves.
5. Sprinkle cheese and grill with the lid covered at medium heat for 10 minutes or until the zucchini are tender. Serve.

Serving suggestion: Serve the stuffed zucchini with charred pork chops.

Variation Tip: use another cheese of choice

Nutrition-Per Serving:
Calories 186| Fat 10g |Sodium 553 mg | Carbs 7g | Fiber 3 g | Sugar 4 g | Protein 9g

Smoked Vegetables

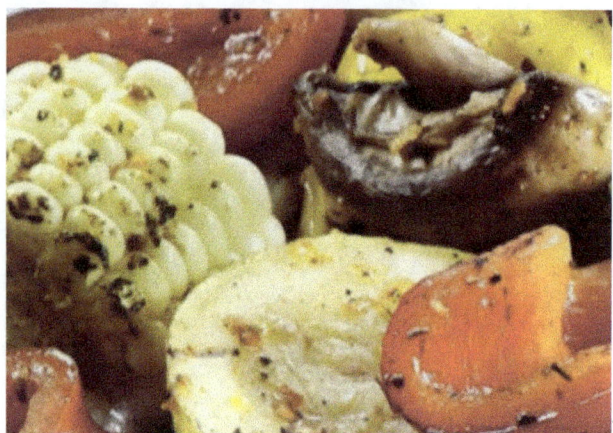

Prep Time: 20 minutes
Cook Time: 15 minutes
Serves: 6

Ingredients:

- 1 ear corn, cut into pieces
- 1 yellow squash, cut into ½ inch pieces
- 1 red onion wedges
- 1 green pepper, cut into strips
- 1 red pepper, cut into strips
- 1 yellow pepper, cut into strips
- 1 cup mushrooms, cut into halves
- 2 tablespoons oil
- 2 tablespoons chicken seasoning

Preparation:

1. Preheat your Pit Boss Wood Pellet Grill to 180 degrees F for 10 minutes.
2. Toss all the vegetables with oil and seasoning.
3. Transfer them to a grill basket or thread onto skewers
4. Grill for 12 minutes while turning occasionally or until the veggies are tender.
5. Serve and enjoy.

Serving suggestion: serve smoked vegetables with smoked chicken thighs.

Variation Tip: use dried herbs for seasoning

Nutrition-Per Serving:
Calories 309| Fat 3g |Sodium 244 mg | Carbs 20g | Fiber 6 g | Sugar 3 g | Protein 34g

Smoked Mushrooms

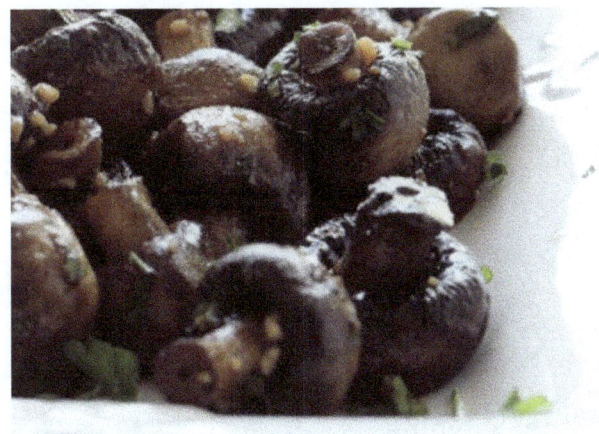

Prep Time: 15 minutes
Cook Time: 45minutes
Serves: 4

Ingredients:

- 4 cups whole Portobello mushrooms
- 1 tablespoon oil
- 1 tablespoon onion powder
- 1 tablespoon granulated garlic
- 1 tablespoon salt
- 1 tablespoon black pepper
- Bread slices and chopped parsley

Preparation:

1. Mix all the ingredients in a bowl until well combined.
2. Fire up your Pit Boss Wood Pellet Grill to 180 degrees F.
3. Smoke the mushrooms for 30 minutes.
4. Remove the mushrooms from the grill and raise the temperature to 500 degrees F.
5. Place the mushroom on the grill and cook for 15 minutes.
6. Serve the mushrooms with bread slices and top with parsley.

Serving suggestion: serve smoked mushroom with avocado sauce topping.

Variation Tip: use cayenne pepper

Nutrition-Per Serving:
Calories 79| Fat 4g |Sodium 1768 mg | Carbs 9g | Fiber 4 g | Sugar 3 g | Protein 4g

Grilled Zucchini Chips

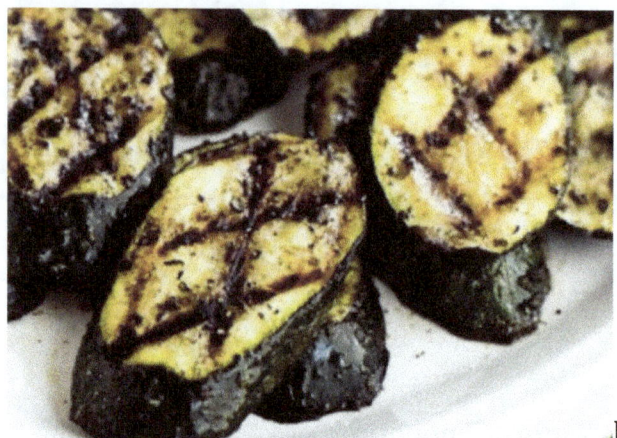

Prep Time: 5 minutes
Cook Time: 10 minutes
Serves: 4

Ingredients:

4 zucchinis, cut into thin slices
2 tablespoons oil
1 tablespoon sherry vinegar
2 thyme leaves, pulled
Salt and pepper to taste

Preparation:

1. Add all the ingredients in a resalable bag then shake to mix.
2. Preheat the Pit Boss Wood Pellet Grill to 350 degrees F.
3. Place the zucchini on the grill grate with the cut side down.
4. Grill the zucchini for about 4 minutes on each side.
5. Serve and enjoy.

Serving suggestion: serve the zucchini chips with roasted chicken.

Variation Tip: use sherry cooking wine in place of sherry vinegar.

Nutrition-Per Serving:
Calories 98| Fat 7g |Sodium 1 mg | Carbs 7g | Fiber 0.5 g | Sugar 1 g | Protein 2g

Roasted Cauliflower with Garlic Parmesan Butter

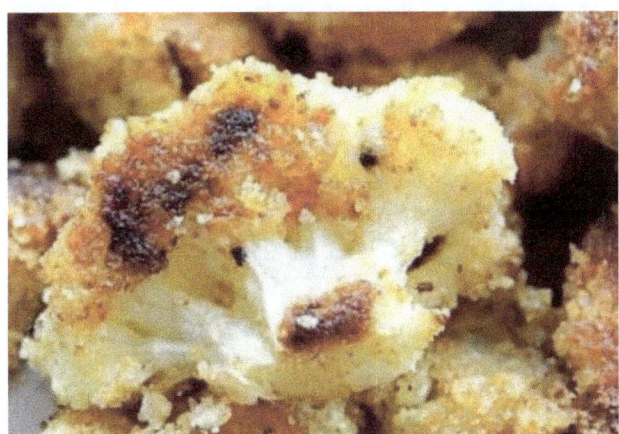

Prep Time: 15 minutes
Cook Time: 45 minutes
Serves: 4

Ingredients:

- 1 cauliflower head
- ¼ cup oil
- Salt and pepper to taste
- ½ cup melted butter
- ¼ cup parmesan cheese
- 2 minced garlic cloves
- ½ tablespoons chopped parsley

Preparation:

1. Fire up your Pit Boss Wood Pellet Grill to 450 degrees F.
2. Coat the cauliflower with oil then season it with salt and pepper.
3. Place the cauliflower in a skillet then place it in the grill grate. Cook for 25 minutes.
4. Meanwhile mix butter, cheese, garlic, and parsley in a bowl.
5. Brush the cauliflower with the butter mixture and cook for 20 minutes.
6. Serve and enjoy.

Serving suggestion: Serve the cauliflower with beef stew.

Variation Tip: use fresh or dried herbs for seasoning.

Nutrition-Per Serving:
Calories 373| Fat 38g |Sodium 316 mg | Carbs 6g | Fiber 2 g | Sugar 2 g | Protein 4g

Smoked Cheddar Cheese

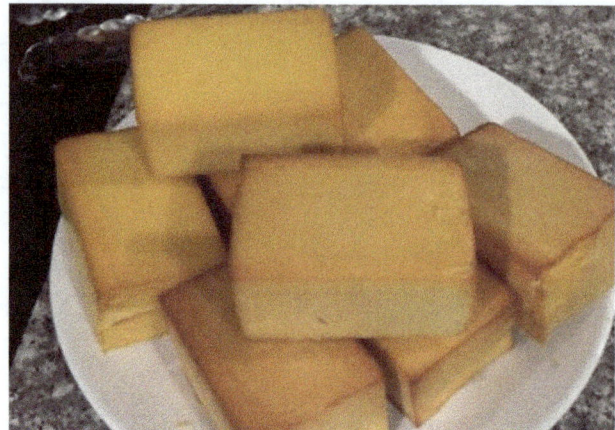

Prep Time: 5 minutes
Cook Time: 2 hours
Serves: 8

Ingredients:

- 2 Pounds cheddar cheese block

Preparation:

1. Fire up your Pit Boss Wood Pellet Grill to 180 degrees F.
2. Fill a deep oven tray with ice and place a wire rack on top.
3. Place the cheese on the wire rack.
4. Place the tray on the grill grate and smoke the cheese for 1 hour.
5. Flip the cheese and add more ice then smoke for an additional 1 hour.
6. Remove the cheese from the grill and wrap it with parchment paper. Refrigerate for 2 days.
7. Serve the cheese on its own or in sandwiches.

Serving suggestion: serve smoked cheddar cheese with favourite cracker and pickled vegetables.

Variation Tip: use frozen cheddar cheese.

Nutrition-Per Serving:
Calories 200| Fat 10g |Sodium 1250 mg | Carbs 12g | Fiber 0 g | Sugar 8 g | Protein 15g

Grilled Asparagus and Honey-Glazed Carrots

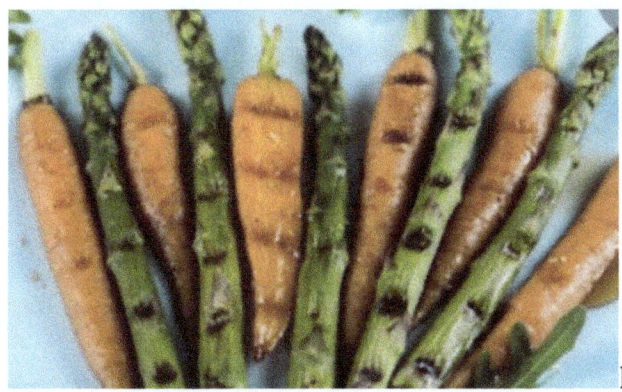

Prep Time: 15 minutes
Cook Time: 35 minutes
Serves: 4

Ingredients:

- 1 bunch asparagus, trimmed
- 2 tablespoons oil
- Salt to taste
- 1 Pound carrots cut into halves lengthwise
- 2 tablespoons honey

Preparation:

1. In a bowl add asparagus, oil, and salt and toss to coat.
2. In a separate bowl add carrots, honey, and salt then toss to coat.
3. Fire up your Pit Boss Wood Pellet Grill to 350 degrees F.
4. Place the carrots on the grill and cook for 15 minutes.
5. Add the asparagus to the grill and cook for 15 minutes.
6. Serve and enjoy.

Serving suggestion: serve grilled asparagus with honey glazed carrots with goat cheese.

Variation Tip: Add garlic powder and onion powder

Nutrition-Per Serving:
Calories 161| Fat 7g |Sodium 81 mg | Carbs 24g | Fiber 6 g | Sugar 16 g | Protein 4g

Pit Boss Wood Pellet Smoked Eggs

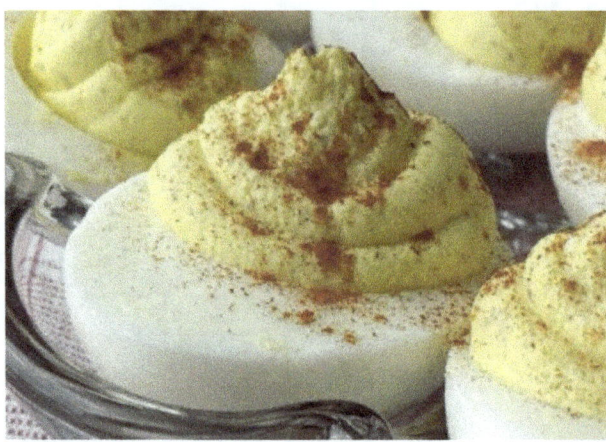

Prep Time: 15 minutes
Cook Time: 30 minutes
Serves: 4

Ingredients:

- 7 hard-boiled eggs, peeled
- 3 tablespoons mayonnaise
- 3 tablespoons diced chives
- 1 tablespoon brown mustard
- 1 tablespoon apple cider vinegar
- 1 tablespoon hot sauce
- Salt and pepper to taste
- ¼ tablespoons paprika
- Parsley leaves

Preparation:

1. Fire up the pellet grill to 180 degrees F.
2. Place the eggs on the grill and smoke for 30 minutes.
3. Remove the eggs from the grill and allow them to cool.
4. Add the egg yolks, mayonnaise, chives, mustard, vinegar, hot sauce, salt, and pepper in a gallon zip bag.
5. Knead the ingredients in the bag until they are smooth.
6. Make a small cut at the corner of the bag and squeeze the egg yolk into egg white.
7. Top the devilled eggs with paprika and parsley.
8. Serve and enjoy.

Serving suggestion: serve these devilled eggs with a cup of coffee.

Variation Tip: Use old bay instead of salt and pepper.

Nutrition-Per Serving:

Calories 288| Fat 22g |Sodium 342 mg | Carbs 4g | Fiber 0.7 g | Sugar 2 g | Protein 17g

FISH AND SEAFOOD RECIPES

Grilled Teriyaki Salmon

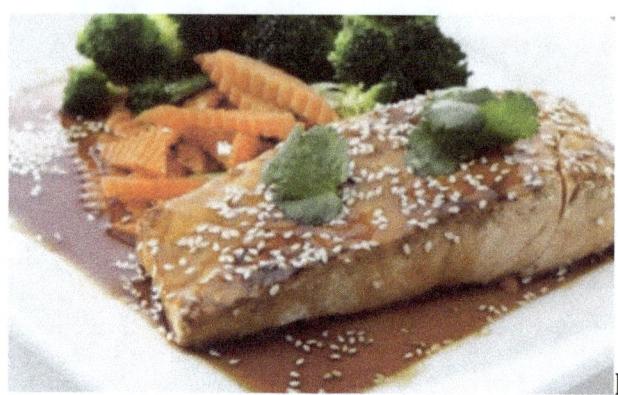

Prep Time: 10 minutes
Cook Time: 20 minutes
Serves: 4

Ingredients:

- 1 salmon fillet
- ⅛ cup oil
- ½ tablespoons salt
- ¼ tablespoons pepper
- ¼ tablespoons garlic salt
- ¼ cup butter, sliced
- ¼ cup teriyaki sauce
- 1 tablespoon sesame seeds

Preparation:

1. Preheat your Pit Boss Wood Pellet Grill to 400 degrees F.
2. Place the salmon fillet in a foil sheet then drizzle it with oil then sprinkle the seasonings and place butter on top.
3. Place the foil sheet in the grill and cook for 8 minutes.
4. Open the grill and brush with sauce and continue to cook for an additional 5 minutes or until the internal temperature reaches 145 degrees F.
5. Remove from the grill and sprinkle with sesame seeds. Serve.

Serving suggestion: serve teriyaki salmon with fried rice.

Variation Tip: add seasonings of choice.

Nutrition-Per Serving:
Calories 296| Fat 25g |Sodium 1179 mg | Carbs 3g | Fiber 0 g | Sugar 3 g | Protein 14g

Grilled Togarashi Salmon

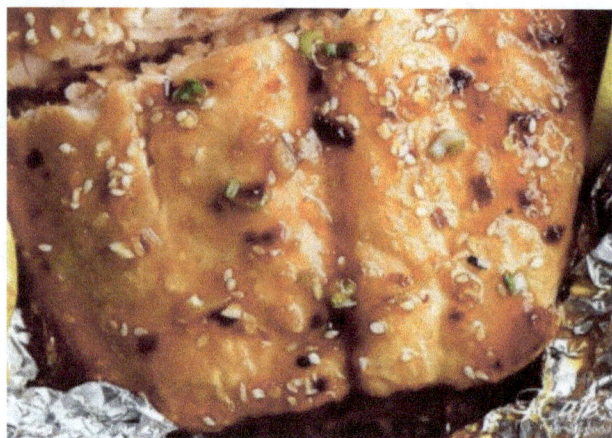

Prep Time: 5 minutes
Cook Time: 20 minutes
Serves: 3

Ingredients:

- 1 salmon fillet
- ¼ cup oil
- ½ tablespoons salt
- 1 tablespoon Togarashi seasoning

Preparation:

1. Preheat your Pit Boss Wood Pellet Grill to 400 degrees F.
2. Place the salmon fillet on a sheet foil with the skin side down.
3. Rub oil then sprinkle salt and Togarashi seasoning on the fillet.
4. Bake in the preheated grill for 20 minutes or until the internal temperature reaches 145 degrees F.
5. Serve immediately.

Serving suggestion: Serve Togarashi salmon with white rice.

Variation Tip: Adjust Togarashi seasoning to your liking.

Nutrition-Per Serving:
Calories 119| Fat 10g |Sodium 433 mg | Carbs 0g | Fiber 0 g | Sugar 0 g | Protein 6g

Grilled Prawn skewers

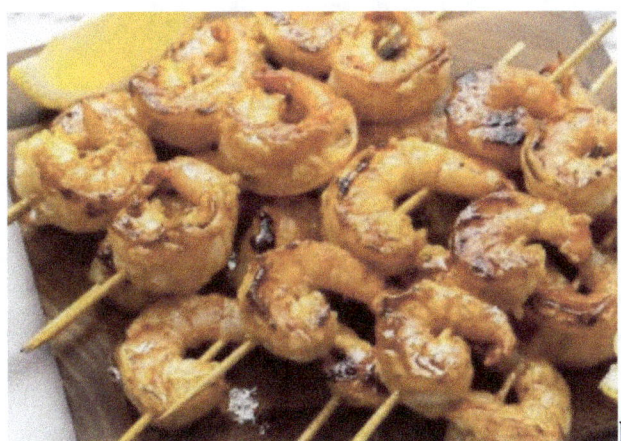

Prep Time: 10 minutes
Cook Time: 10 minutes
Serves: 6

Ingredients:

- 2 Pounds prawns, clean
- 2 tablespoons oil
- Salt and pepper to taste

Preparation:

1. Preheat your Pit Boss Wood Pellet Grill to 400 degrees F.
2. Skewer the prawns on soaked skewers. Brush them with oil then sprinkle with salt and pepper.
3. Place the skewers on the grill grate and cook for 5 minutes per side.
4. Serve and enjoy.

Serving suggestion: serve prawn skewers with cooked veggies.

Variation Tip: Add cayenne pepper in place of pepper.

Nutrition-Per Serving:
Calories 221| Fat 7g |Sodium 1481 mg | Carbs 2g | Fiber 0 g | Sugar 0 g | Protein 34g

Grilled Bacon Wrapped Scallops

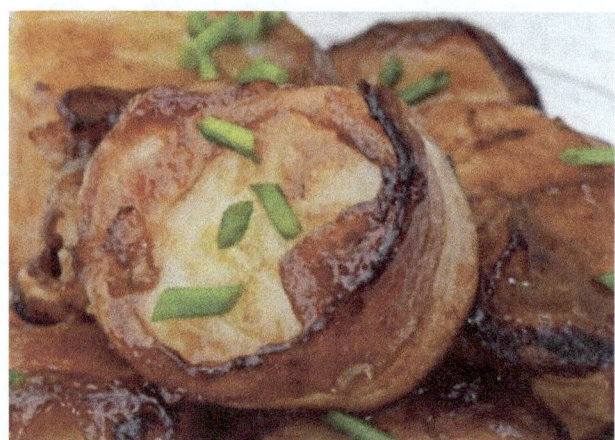

Prep Time: 15 minutes
Cook Time: 20 minutes
Serves: 8

Ingredients:

- 1 Pound scallops
- ½ Pounds bacon
- Salt to taste

Preparation:

1. Preheat your Pit Boss Wood Pellet Grill to 350 degrees F.
2. Pat your scallops with a paper towel until they don't have any moisture.
3. Wrap each scallop with a bacon piece and secure it with a toothpick.
4. Lay them on the grill with the bacon side down. Cook for 7 minutes while rotating them occasionally.
5. Serve and enjoy.

Serving suggestion: Serve these bacon-wrapped scallops with red pepper aioli.

Variation Tip: Use turkey bacon instead of regular bacon.

Nutrition-Per Serving:
Calories 261| Fat 14g |Sodium 1238 mg | Carbs 5g | Fiber 0 g | Sugar 0 g | Protein 28g

Grilled Lobster Tail

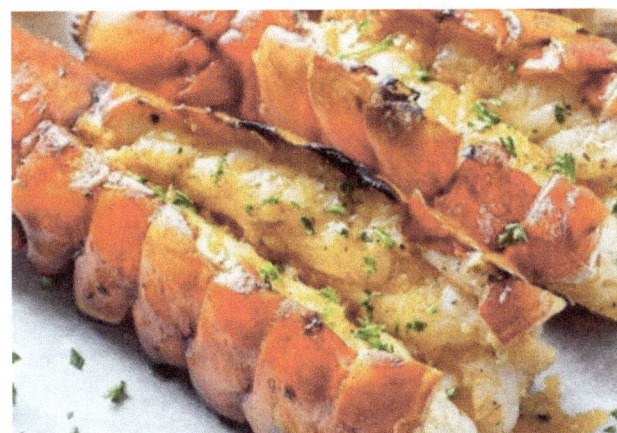

Prep Time: 10 minutes
Cook Time: 15 minutes
Serves: 2

Ingredients:

- 10 Ounces lobster tail
- ¼ tablespoons old bay seasoning
- ¼ tablespoons salt
- 2 tablespoons butter
- 1 tablespoon fresh parsley

Preparation:

1. Preheat your Pit Boss Wood Pellet Grill to 450 degrees F.
2. Slice the lobster tail with a knife and season with old bay seasoning and salt.
3. Place the tail on the grill with the meat side down. Cook for 15 minutes or until the internal temperature reaches 140 degrees F.
4. Remove from the grill and drizzle with butter. Sprinkle parsley and serve.

Serving suggestion: serve grilled lobster tails with grilled cheddar bay biscuits.

Variation Tip: Use fresh thyme in place of fresh parsley.

Nutrition-Per Serving:
Calories 305| Fat 14g |Sodium 684 mg | Carbs 5 g | Fiber 0 g | Sugar 0 g | Protein 38g

Pit Boss Wood Pellet Grill Grilled Lingcod

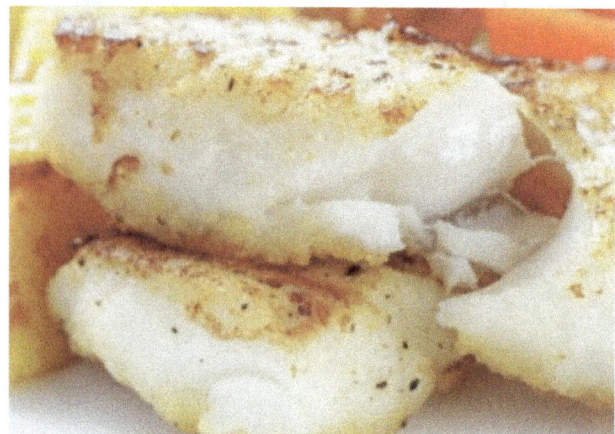

Prep Time: 10 minutes
Cook Time: 15 minutes
Serves: 6

Ingredients:

- 2 Pounds lingcod fillets
- ½ tablespoons salt
- ½ tablespoons pepper
- ¼ tablespoons cayenne
- Lemon slices

Preparation:

1. Fire up your Pit Boss Wood Pellet Grill to 375 degrees F.
2. Place the lingcod fillet on a foil and season it with salt, pepper, cayenne pepper, and top with lemon slices.
3. Place in the grill and cook for 15 minutes or until the internal temperature reaches 145 degrees F.
4. Serve and enjoy.

Serving suggestion: serve grilled lingcod with roasted potatoes.

Variation Tip: Use ground ginger and cayenne pepper.

Nutrition-Per Serving:
Calories 245| Fat 2g |Sodium 442 mg | Carbs 2 g | Fiber 1 g | Sugar 1 g | Protein 52g

Smoked Salmon

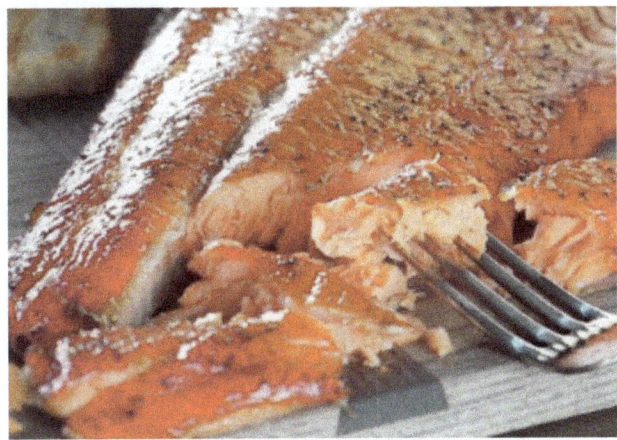

Prep Time: 15 minutes
Cook Time: 4 hours
Serves: 12

Ingredients:

- 4 cups water
- 1 cup brown sugar
- ⅓ cup salt
- 6 Pounds salmon fillet, skin on
- 4 tablespoons maple syrup
- Lettuce leaves

Preparation:

1. Prepare brine by mixing water, sugar, and salt until all the sugar dissolves.
2. Add the salmon and the brine in a ziplock bag and refrigerate for 10 hours.
3. Rinse the salmon and dry it with a paper towel.
4. Fire up your Pit Boss Wood Pellet Grill to 180 degrees F.
5. Place the salmon on the grill and smoke it for 4 hours. Brush the salmon with maple syrup after every 1 hour of smoking.
6. Serve the salmon with lettuce leaves.

Serving suggestion: serve smoked salmon with cream cheese.

Variation Tip: Use sliced cucumber instead of lettuce leaves.

Nutrition-Per Serving:
Calories 101| Fat 2g |Sodium 3131 mg | Carbs 16 g | Fiber 0 g | Sugar 16 g | Protein 4g

Grilled Shrimp Scampi

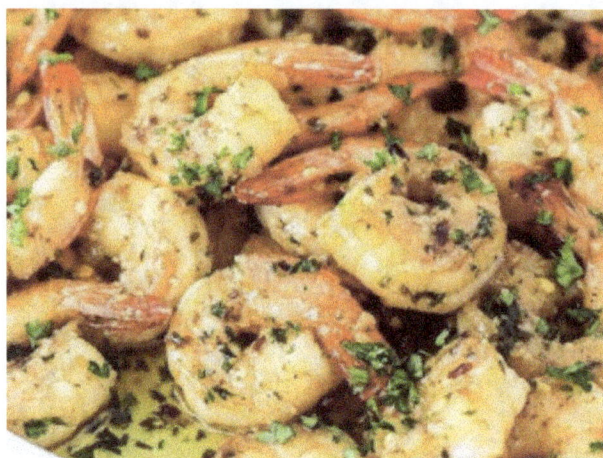

Prep Time: 5 minutes
Cook Time: 10 minutes
Serves: 4

Ingredients:

- ½ cup melted butter
- ¼ cup dry white wine
- ½ tablespoons freshly chopped garlic
- 1 tablespoon lemon juice
- 1 Pound shrimp, peeled and deveined
- ½ tablespoons garlic powder
- ½ tablespoons salt
- Toppings: chopped parsley

Preparation:

1. Fire up your Pit Boss Wood Pellet Grill to 400 degrees F. Set a pan on the grill.
2. Add butter, wine, chopped garlic and lemon juice to the pan and heat for 4 minutes.
3. Season the shrimp with garlic powder and salt then place them in the pan.
4. Cook the shrimp with the lid closed for 10 minutes.
5. Serve the shrimp and top with parsley.

Serving suggestion: serve this grilled shrimp scampi with pasta.

Variation Tip: Use chopped shallots

Nutrition-Per Serving:
Calories 298| Fat 24g |Sodium 1091 mg | Carbs 2 g | Fiber 0 g | Sugar 0 g | Protein 16g

Grilled Scallops

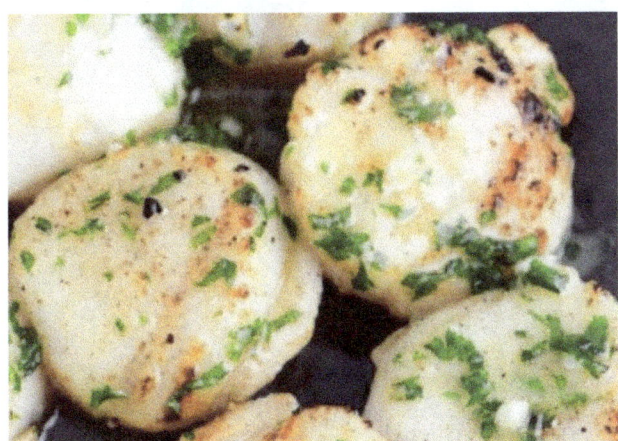

Prep Time: 5 minutes
Cook Time: 15 minutes
Serves: 4

Ingredients:

- 2 Pounds sea scallops
- ½ tablespoons garlic salt
- 1 tablespoon kosher salt
- A dash of white pepper
- 4 tablespoons salted butter
- 1 lemon, juiced

Preparation:

1. Preheat your Pit Boss Wood Pellet Grill to 400 degrees F with a pan set inside.
2. Season the scallops with garlic salt, kosher salt, and pepper.
3. Add the butter and scallops to the pan and close the lid.
4. Cook the scallops for 15 minutes, flipping them halfway through cooking.
5. Remove the scallops from the grill and add the lemon juice.
6. Serve and enjoy.

Serving suggestion: serve these grilled scallops with basmati rice.

Variation Tip: Use black pepper or cayenne pepper in place of white pepper.

Nutrition-Per Serving:
Calories 177 | Fat 7g | Sodium 1430 mg | Carbs 6 g | Fiber 0 g | Sugar 0 g | Protein 23g

Grilled Salmon Sandwich

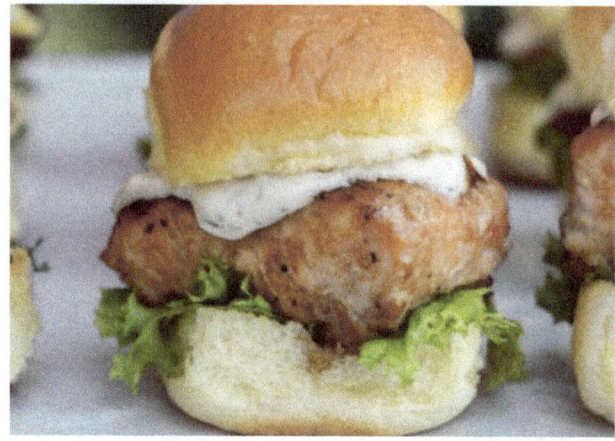

Prep Time: 10 minutes
Cook Time: 15 minutes
Serves: 4

Ingredients:

For the Sandwich:
- 4 salmon fillets
- 1 tablespoon oil
- Fin and feather rub
- 1 tablespoon salt
- 4 toasted buns, cut into halves
- Basil leaves
- 1 red onion, cut into rings
- 1 lemon cut into wedges

For the Dill Aioli:
- ½ cup mayonnaise
- ½ tablespoons lemon zest
- 2 tablespoons lemon juice
- ¼ tablespoons salt
- ½ tablespoons fresh dill, minced

Preparation:

1. Fire up your Pit Boss Wood Pellet Grill to 425 degrees F.
2. Coat the salmon fillets with oil then season them with fin and feather rub and salt.
3. Place the fillets on the grill grates and cook for 7 minutes on each side.
4. Meanwhile, mix all the aioli ingredients in a bowl until they are well combined.

5. Remove the fillets from the grill and let them rest for 5 minutes.
6. Assemble the sandwich. Top each of the 4 buns with basil leaves then layer the salmon fillet. Place the onion rings on the fillet and pour the aioli over the sandwich. Cover the sandwich with the remaining buns.
7. Serve the sandwich immediately with lemon wedges.

Serving suggestion: Serve the grilled salmon sandwich with grilled scalloped potatoes.

Variation Tip: Use coleslaw in place of lettuce.

Nutrition-Per Serving:
Calories 852 | Fat 54g |Sodium 1268 mg | Carbs 30 g | Fiber 2 g | Sugar 5 g | Protein 57g

Smoked Buffalo Shrimp

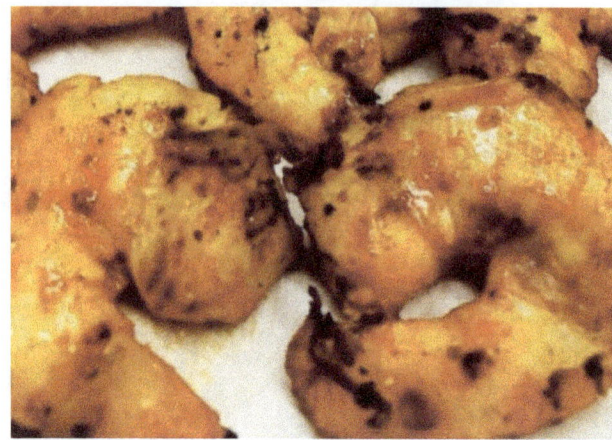

Prep Time: 10 minutes
Cook Time: 5 minutes
Serves: 6

Ingredients:

- 1 Pound shrimp, peeled and deveined
- ½ tablespoons salt
- ¼ tablespoons garlic powder
- ¼ tablespoons onion powder
- ½ cup buffalo sauce

Preparation:

1. Fire up your Pit Boss Wood Pellet Grill to 450 degrees F.
2. Season the shrimp with salt, garlic powder, and onion powder.
3. Place the shrimp on the grill grate and cook for 3 minutes on each side.
4. Remove the shrimp from the grill and toss in buffalo sauce.
5. Serve and enjoy.

Serving suggestion: serve the smoked buffalo shrimp with green onions toppings.

Variation Tip: use homemade buffalo sauce and additional herbs of choice.

Nutrition-Per Serving:
Calories 108 | Fat 1g |Sodium 917 mg | Carbs 10 g | Fiber 0.3 g | Sugar 7 g | Protein 15g

SNACK AND APPETIZERS RECIPES

Baked Bacon Wrapped Jalapeno Poppers

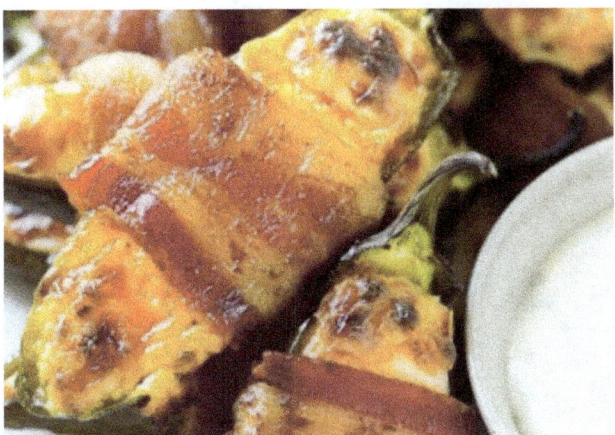

Prep Time: 10 minutes
Cook Time: 25 minutes
Serves: 4

Ingredients:
- 6 jalapenos
- 4oz cream cheese
- ½ cup cheddar cheese, shredded
- 1 tablespoon veggie rub
- 12 slices thinly cut bacon

Preparation:
1. Preheat your Pit Boss Wood Pellet Grill to 375 degrees F.
2. Slice the jalapenos lengthwise and scrape out the seeds and membrane. Set aside.
3. In a mixing bowl, mix cream cheese, cheddar cheese, veggie rub until well mixed.
4. Fill the jalapeno halves with the mixture then wrap each with a bacon slice.
5. Grill for 20 minutes or until the jalapenos are soft and the bacon is crispy.

Serving suggestion: serve these bacon-wrapped jalapenos with ranch dressing.

Variation Tip: Add chopped mushrooms.

Nutrition-Per Serving:
Calories 3231 | Fat 15g | Sodium 994 mg | Carbs 5 g | Fiber 0.7 g | Sugar 2 g | Protein 19g

Grilled Watermelon Wedges

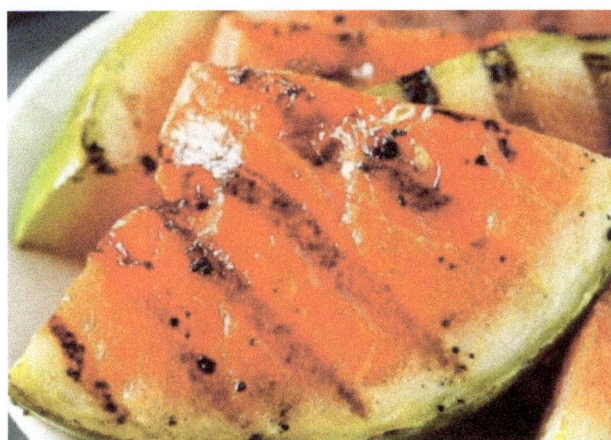

Prep Time: 10 minutes
Cook Time: 15 minutes
Serves: 2

Ingredients:

- ½ watermelon, cut into wedges
- 2 tablespoons oil
- 2 tablespoons salt
- ¼ tablespoons red pepper flakes
- 2 limes juice

Preparation:

1. Preheat your Pit Boss Wood Pellet Grill to 500 degrees F for 15 minutes with the lid closed.
2. Brush the watermelon wedges with oil then place them on grill grates.
3. Grill for 15 minutes while flipping them halfway through the cooking session.
4. Meanwhile, mix salt and pepper flakes until well combined.
5. Remove lemon from the grill, squeeze lime juice and sprinkle with the salt mixture.
6. Serve.

Serving suggestion: serve the grilled watermelon with blue cheese and prosciutto strips toppings.

Variation Tip: use chopped basil and cilantro.

Nutrition-Per Serving:
Calories 131 | Fat 14g |Sodium 1141 mg | Carbs 3 g | Fiber 0.3 g | Sugar 1g | Protein 1g

Roasted Sweet Potatoes

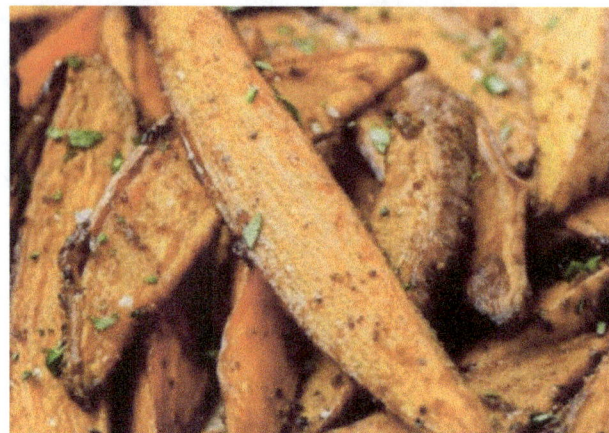

Prep Time: 15 minutes
Cook Time: 30 minutes
Serves: 4

Ingredients:

- 4 sweet potatoes, wedges
- 3 tablespoons oil
- 1 tablespoon salt
- 1 tablespoon black pepper
- 1 cup mayonnaise
- 2 chipotle peppers in adobo sauce
- 2 limes juice

Preparation:

1. Preheat your Pit Boss Wood Pellet Grill to 400 degrees F for 15 minutes with the lid closed.
2. Toss the sweet potatoes with oil, salt, and pepper. Spread them on a sheet pan.
3. Place the sheet pan on the grill grate and cook for 30 minutes while stirring occasionally or until crispy.
4. Meanwhile, mix mayo, peppers, and juice in a blender. Blend until smooth.
5. Serve the sweet potato fries with the sauce.

Serving suggestion: serve the roasted sweet potatoes with grilled chicken thighs.

Variation Tip: Use lemon juice in place of lime juice.

Nutrition-Per Serving:
Calories 323 | Fat 30g |Sodium 1141 mg | Carbs 15 g | Fiber 3g | Sugar 4g | Protein 1g

Smoked Sweet and Spicy Cashew

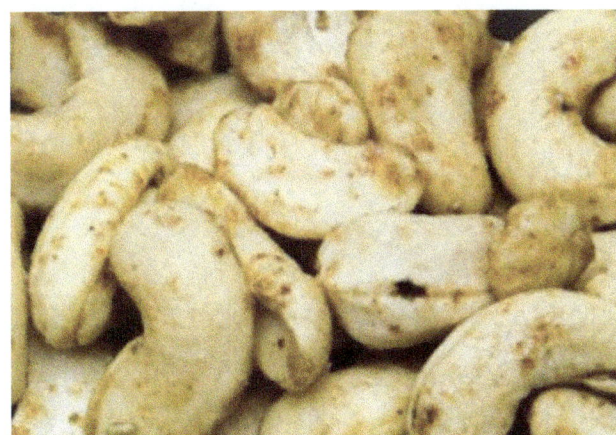

Prep Time: 5 minutes
Cook Time: 1 hour
Serves: 6

Ingredients:
- 3 tablespoons sambal oelek
- 1 lemon, zested
- ½ tablespoons rosemary, chopped
- 1 tablespoon red pepper flakes
- ¼ tablespoons cayenne powder
- 1 Pound cashews

Preparation:
1. Preheat your Pit Boss Wood Pellet Grill to 225 degrees F for 15 minutes with the lid closed.
2. In a mixing bowl, mix sambal oelek, lemon zest, rosemary, pepper flakes, and cayenne powder.
3. Pour the mixture over cashews and mix well.
4. Spread the cashews on a sheet pan and place the sheet pan on the grill grates.
5. Cook for 1 hour while stirring occasionally. Let cool before serving.

Serving suggestion: serve the smoked cashews with a cool drink.

Variation Tip: Use coriander and smoked paprika

Nutrition-Per Serving:
Calories 439 | Fat 35g | Sodium 6 mg | Carbs 26 g | Fiber 6g | Sugar 2g | Protein 12g

Smoked Nut Mix

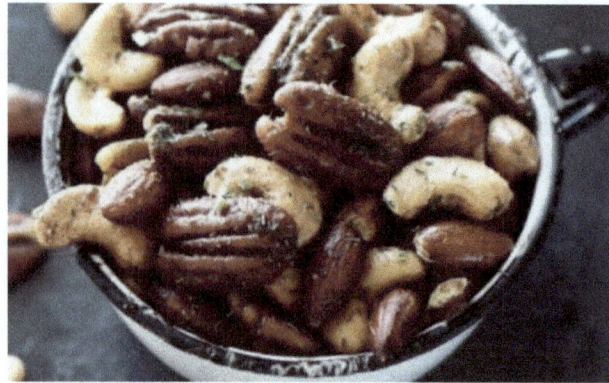

Prep Time: 15 minutes
Cook Time: 20 minutes
Serves: 8

Ingredients:

- 3 cups mixed nuts (almond, pecans, cashews, walnuts)
- 1½ tablespoons brown sugar
- 1 tablespoon dried dill
- ½ tablespoons dried chives
- ¼ tablespoons cayenne powder
- ¼ tablespoons mustard powder
- 1 tablespoon oil

Preparation:

1. Fire up your Pit Boss Wood Pellet Grill to 250 degrees F.
2. Add all the ingredients to a bowl and toss to mix.
3. Transfer the mixed nuts to a baking sheet lined with parchment paper.
4. Place the baking sheet on the grill and cook the nuts for 20 minutes.
5. Remove the nuts from the grill and serve.

Serving suggestion: serve the smoked nut mix with apple and pineapple slices.

Variation Tip: Use chipotle powder in place of cayenne powder.

Nutrition-Per Serving:
Calories 321 | Fat 28g | Sodium 6 mg | Carbs 12 g | Fiber 6g | Sugar 2g | Protein 11g

Smoked Cinnamon Almonds

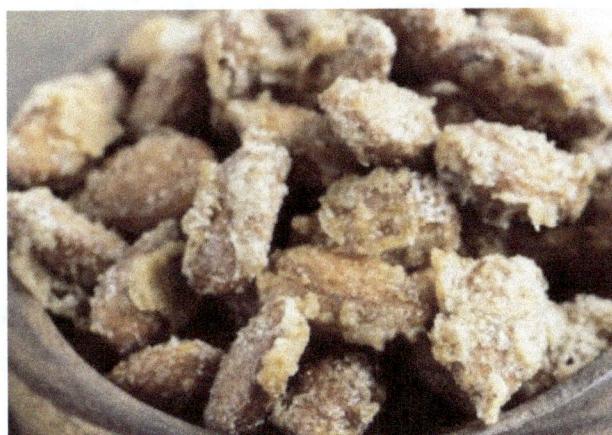

Prep Time: 15 minutes
Cook Time: 1 hour 30 minutes
Serves: 4

Ingredients:

1 egg white
2 tablespoons vanilla extract
2 cups unsalted almonds
1 cup brown sugar
1 tablespoon cinnamon
¾ tablespoons salt
½ tablespoons nutmeg
¼ tablespoons ground ginger

Preparation:

1. Fire up your Pit Boss Wood Pellet Grill to 225 degrees F.
2. In a bowl mix the egg white and vanilla extract.
3. Add the almonds to the egg white mixture and toss to coat.
4. In a separate bowl mix sugar, cinnamon, salt, nutmeg, and ginger.
5. Pour the sugar mixture over the almonds and toss to mix.
6. Transfer the almonds to a baking sheet lined with parchment paper.
7. Place the baking sheet on the grill and smoke for 1½ hour.
8. Let the almonds cool for 30 minutes then break them up.
9. Serve and enjoy.

Serving suggestion: serve the cinnamon almonds with Brussels sprouts salad.

Variation Tip: Use white sugar in place of brown sugar.

Nutrition-Per Serving:

Calories 607 | Fat 44g |Sodium 1324 mg | Carbs 42 g | Fiber 9g | Sugar 28g | Protein 18g

Pit Boss Wood Pellet Grill Smoked Olives

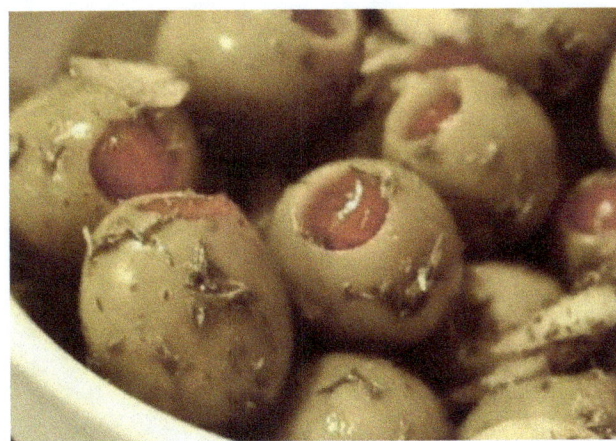

Prep Time: 15 minutes
Cook Time: 2 hours
Serves: 6

Ingredients:

- 2 cup green olives
- 2 tablespoons oil
- 2 tablespoons white wine
- 2 minced garlic cloves
- ¾ tablespoons dried rosemary
- ¼ tablespoons red pepper flakes

Preparation:

1. Fire up your wood pellet grill to 220 degrees F.
2. Mix all the ingredients in a heavy-duty aluminium foil that has been moulded into a tray.
3. Place the olives on the grill and cook for 2 hours.
4. Serve and enjoy.

Serving suggestion: serve the grilled olives with your favourite cheese

Variation Tip: use more herbs of choice.

Nutrition-Per Serving:
Calories 64 | Fat 6g |Sodium 15 mg | Carbs 3 g | Fiber 1g | Sugar 1g | Protein 1g

DESSERT RECIPES

Grilled Apricot with Gelato

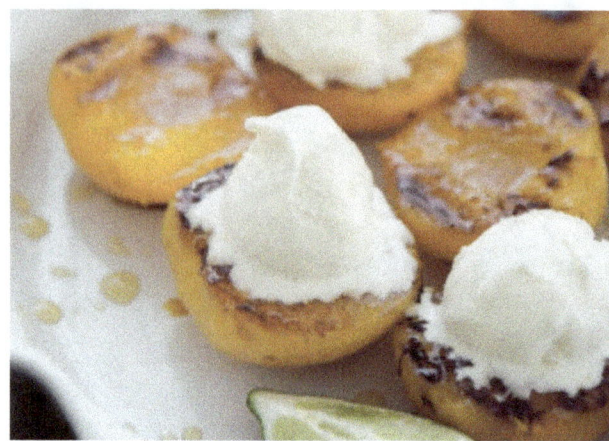

Prep Time: 5 minutes
Cook Time: 5 minutes
Serves: 2

Ingredients:

- 2 apricots, halved
- ¼ cup honey
- 3 tablespoons white sugar
- Gelato for serving

Preparation:

1. Preheat your Pit Boss Wood Pellet Grill to 450 degrees F for 15 minutes with the lid closed.
2. Brush the apricot halves with honey then sprinkle with sugar.
3. Place the apricots on the grill grates cut side down and cook until you see the grill marks.
4. Serve with a scoop of gelato and drizzle with more honey if you like.

Serving suggestion: serve the grilled apricot with ham and arugula.

Variation Tip: Use black sugar in place of white sugar.

Nutrition-Per Serving:
Calories 213 | Fat 0.2g |Sodium 15mg | Carbs 57 g | Fiber 4g | Sugar 49g | Protein 0.1g

Baked Coconut Cookies

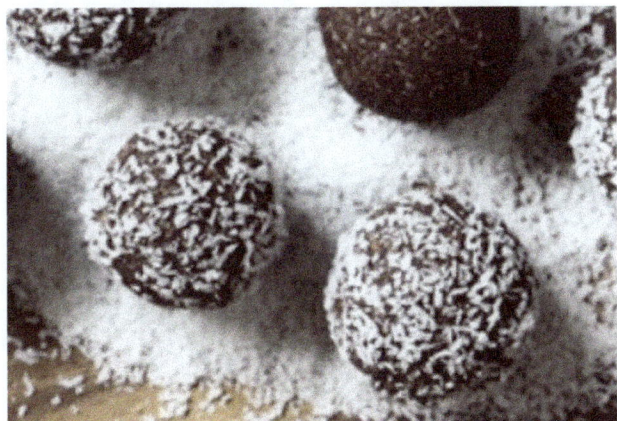

Prep Time: 5 minutes
Cook Time: 15 minutes
Serves: 8

Ingredients:

- 4 eggs
- 4 tablespoons brown sugar
- 1 cup coconut flakes
- 1 pinch salt
- ½ cup chocolate, chopped
- 5 tablespoons butter, melted
- Salt for serving

Preparation:

1. Preheat your Pit Boss Wood Pellet Grill to 375 degrees F for 15 minutes with the lid closed.
2. Line a baking tray with foil.
3. In a mixing bowl, mix eggs, sugar, coconut flakes, salt, chocolate, and butter until well combined.
4. Let the mixture rest for 20 minutes. Spoon the mixture onto a tray and shape them like a circle.
5. Bake in the grill for 15 minutes or until the top is golden brown.
6. Sprinkle it with salt and grated coconut
7. . Enjoy.

Serving suggestion: serve the coconut cookie with caramel apple dip.

Variation Tip: Use granulated sugar in place of brown sugar.

Nutrition-Per Serving:

Calories 209 | Fat 16g | Sodium 152 mg | Carbs 14 g | Fiber 1g | Sugar 10g | Protein 4g

Grilled Peaches and Cream

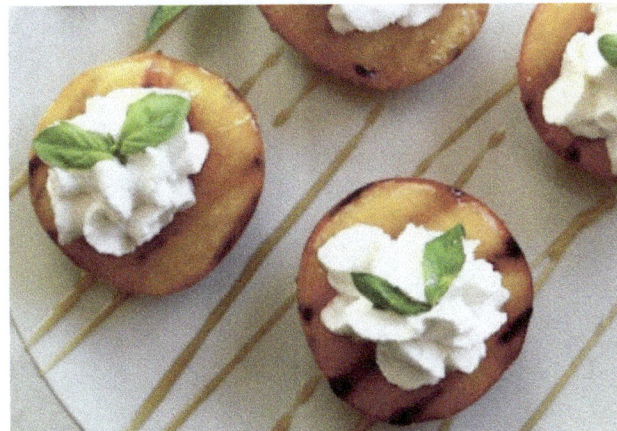

Prep Time: 15 minutes
Cook Time: 8 minutes
Serves: 8

Ingredients:

- 4 peaches, halved
- 2 tablespoons honey
- 1 cup cream cheese
- 1 tablespoon oil

Preparation:

1. Preheat your Pit Boss Wood Pellet Grill to medium heat.
2. Brush the peaches halves with a light coating of oil.
3. Place the peaches on the grill grates with the cut side down. Grill for 5 minutes.
4. Turn the peaches, drizzle with honey and place a dollop of cream cheese on top.
5. Grill for an additional 3 minutes.
6. Serve immediately.

Serving suggestion: serve grilled peaches with fresh berries toppings.

Variation Tip: brown sugar and cinnamon can be added before grilling.

Nutrition-Per Serving:
Calories 139 | Fat 10g |Sodium 135mg | Carbs 12 g | Fiber 1g | Sugar 10g | Protein 2g

Grilled Mango with Coconut Yogurt

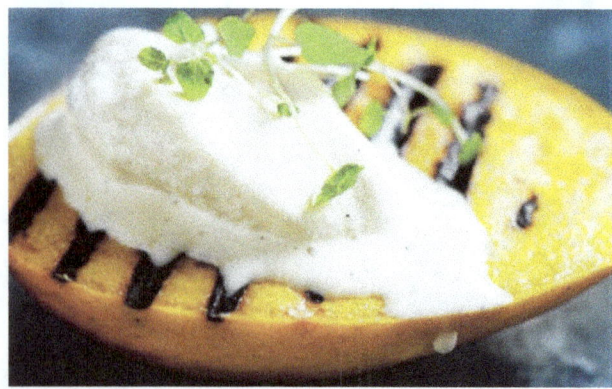

Prep Time: 10 minutes
Cook Time: 15 minutes
Serves: 2

Ingredients:

- 4 ripe mangoes cut into cheeks
- 3 tablespoons maple syrup
- 1 cup coconut yogurt, frozen
- Mint leaves

Preparation:

1. Fire up your Pit Boss Wood Pellet Grill to 500 degrees F.
2. Brush the mango cheeks with maple syrup.
3. Place the mango cheeks on the grill grate and grill for 10 minutes.
4. Top the mango cheeks with 1 spoonful of the yogurt and garnish with mint leaves.
5. Serve and enjoy.

Serving suggestion: serve grilled mango with coconut flakes and lemon zest.

Variation Tip: Use chile powder.

Nutrition-Per Serving:
Calories 500 | Fat 14g | Sodium 132 mg | Carbs 95 g | Fiber 5g | Sugar 49g | Protein 7g

Grilled Blueberry Buckle Coffee Cake

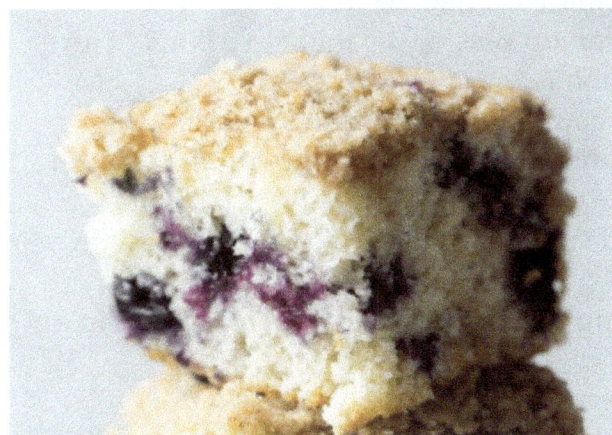

Prep Time: 20 minutes
Cook Time: 45 minutes
Serves: 10

Ingredients:

For the Blueberry Buckle:
- 8 tablespoons softened butter
- ¾ cups granulated sugar
- 1 egg
- 1 tablespoon lemon juice
- 1 tablespoon lemon zest
- 1 tablespoon vanilla extract
- 2 cups all-purpose flour
- ½ tablespoons salt
- 2 tablespoons cinnamon
- 2½ tablespoons baking powder
- ½ cup milk
- 2 cups fresh blueberries

For the Streusel Topping:
- ¾ cups brown sugar
- 1 ¼ cup all-purpose flour
- ¼ tablespoons salt
- ½ tablespoons cinnamon
- 8 tablespoons butter

Preparation:

1. Fire up your Pit Boss Wood Pellet Grill to 375 degrees F.
2. Add butter, sugar, egg, lemon juice, lemon zest, and vanilla to a bowl of an electric mixer and mix until well combined.
3. In a separate bowl sift the flour, salt, cinnamon, and baking powder.
4. Gradually add the flour mixture and milk to the egg mixture until a smooth batter is formed.
5. Pour the batter into a baking pan and spread it evenly. Top the batter with blueberries.
6. Prepare the streusel topping by mixing sugar, flour, salt, and cinnamon in a bowl. Stir in butter until well mixed.
7. Sprinkle the streusels over the blueberries.
8. Place the baking pan on the grill and bake the cake for 45 minutes.
9. Remove the cake from the grill and cool slightly.
10. Serve and enjoy.

Serving suggestion: serve the blueberry buckle coffee cake with a cup of coffee.

Variation Tip: Use frozen blueberries.

Nutrition-Per Serving:

Calories 481 | Fat 20g |Sodium 696 mg | Carbs70 g | Fiber 3g | Sugar 35g | Protein 6g

Grilled Maple Bacon Donuts

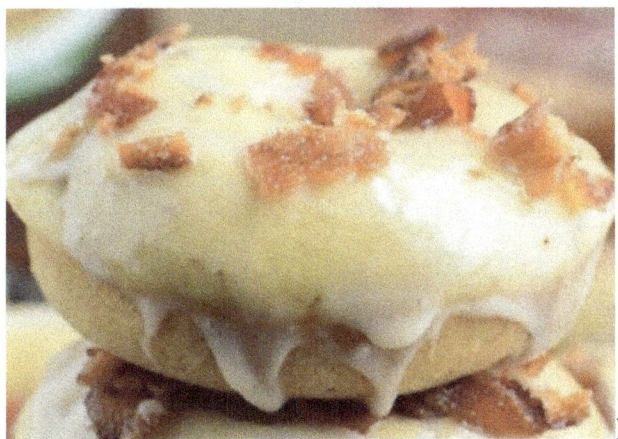

Prep Time: 5 minutes
Cook Time: 15 minutes
Serves: 8

Ingredients:

- 1½ cup powdered sugar
- ¼ cup maple syrup
- 2 tablespoons maple extract
- 2 tablespoons heavy cream
- 2 bacon strips
- 12 glazed yeast doughnuts

Preparation:

1. Preheat your Pit Boss Wood Pellet Grill to 500 degrees F.
2. Add sugar, maple syrup, maple extract to a saucepan and cook on a stovetop at medium-high heat until the mixture comes to a boil.
3. Reduce the heat to low and stir in the heavy cream to the sugar mixture.
4. Place the bacon on the grill grate and grill for 7 minutes.
5. Remove the bacon from the grill and let it cool. Chop into small pieces.
6. Place the doughnuts on the grill and grill them for 5 minutes on each side.
7. Transfer the doughnuts to a serving platter, pour over the glaze, and sprinkle them with bacon.
8. Serve and enjoy.

Serving suggestion: serve maple bacon donuts with a cup of hot chocolate.

Variation Tip: use Greek yogurt in place of heavy cream.

Nutrition-Per Serving:
Calories 491 | Fat 22g |Sodium 321mg | Carbs69 g | Fiber 2g | Sugar 48g | Protein 6g

Grilled Honey Cornbread Cake

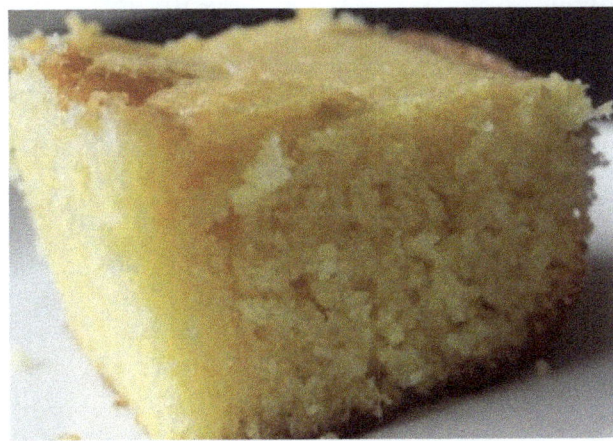

Prep Time: 10 minutes
Cook Time: 40 minutes
Serves: 8

Ingredients:

- ⅔ cup oil
- 2½ cup buttermilk
- 4 eggs, beaten
- 6 tablespoons melted butter
- ½ cup mayonnaise
- 2 tablespoons honey
- 3 cup all-purpose flour
- 2 tablespoons baking powder
- 1 tablespoon salt
- 1 cup cornmeal
- 1½ cup granulated sugar

Preparation:

1. Fire up your Pit Boss Wood Pellet Grill to 350 degrees F.
2. In a bowl mix oil, buttermilk, eggs, 5 tablespoons butter, mayonnaise, and honey until well combined.
3. In a separate bowl mix flour, baking powder, salt, cornmeal, and sugar.
4. Stir in the flour mixture into the egg mixture until a smooth batter is formed.
5. Pour the batter into a baking dish that has been greased with 1 tablespoon of butter.
6. Place the baking dish on the grill grate and cook for 40 minutes.
7. Let the cake rest for 10 minutes before slicing.
8. Serve and enjoy.

Serving suggestion: serve cornbread cake with honey.

Variation Tip: use breadcrumbs in place of cornmeal.

Nutrition-Per Serving:

Calories 701 | Fat 37g |Sodium 1256mg | Carbs79 g | Fiber 2g | Sugar 27g | Protein 14g

CONCLUSION

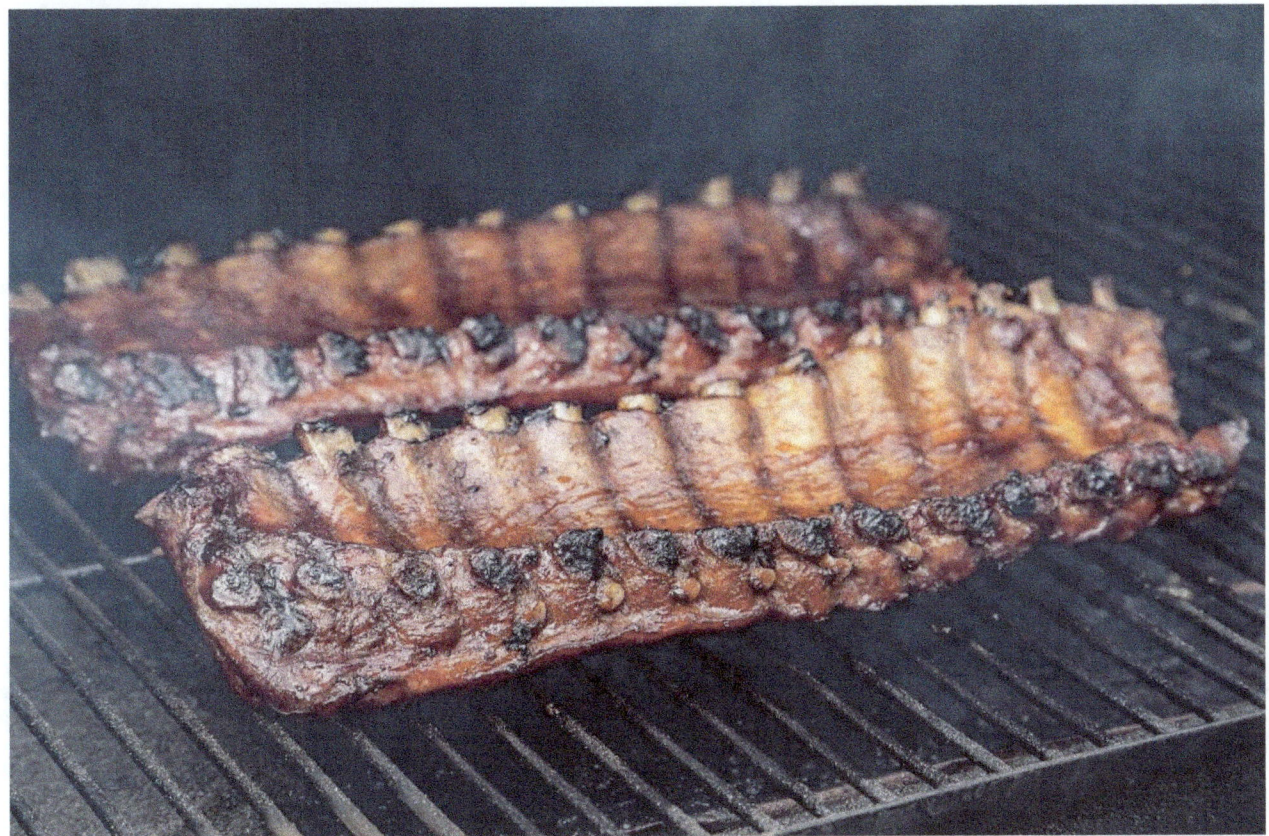

Having gone through an overview of what is the Pit Boss Wood Pellet Grill, some valuable tips, and a plethora of delicious recipes, there is no doubt that it is a must-have for any grillers.

Although using the appliance may prove challenging the first time around, trying a recipe more than once and using different wood pellets flavours will help you achieve blue ribbon cooking.

Last but not least, different models of the pit boss wood pallet are released now and then. Consequently, the different brands will serve you differently. Therefore, shop smartly and purchase a Pit Boss wood pallet that perfectly meets your needs. HAVE FUN!

www.ingramcontent.com/pod-product-compliance
Lightning Source LLC
Chambersburg PA
CBHW081416080526
44589CB00016B/2556